Information Management

The Compliance Guide to the JCAHO Standards

D1716394

Second Edition

Information Management—The Compliance Guide to the JCAHO Standards (**2nd edition**) is published by Opus Communications.

Copyright 1998 by Opus Communications, Inc. Second printing.

All rights reserved. Printed in the United States of America.   5   4   3   2

ISBN: 1-885829-30-2

Opus Communications provides information resources for the health care industry. A listing of our newsletters and books is found in the back of this book.

Opus Communications is not affiliated in any way with the Joint Commission on Accreditation of Healthcare Organizations.

James B. Flanagan, Publisher
Maureen M. Wrinn, Book Editor
Fran Nicholson, Copy Editor
Jean St. Pierre, Design and Layout

Advice given is general and readers should consult professional counsel for specific legal, ethical, or clinical questions.

For more information, contact:

Opus Communications
P.O. Box 1168
Marblehead, MA 01945
Telephone: 800/753-0131 or 781/639-1872
Fax: 781/639-2982
E-Mail: Customer_service@opuscomm.com

Visit the Opus Communications World Wide Web site: http://www.opuscomm.com

 All text pages are printed on recycled paper.

About the Authors

Jennifer I. Cofer, RRA, is publisher of *Medical Records Briefing*. She has served as president of the American Health Information Management Association (formerly the American Medical Record Association) and as the organization's director of communications and professional practices. Ms. Cofer's professional activities include serving as chair of the Mental Health Records Section of the American Medical Records Association and as a member of the advisory board of the *Journal of the American Association for Medical Transcription*.

Hugh P. Greeley is chair of The Greeley Company, and a partner in The Credentialling Institute. He is a contributing editor to *Briefings on JCAHO* and *The Credentialing Resource Center*, and a board member of Incarnate Word Hospital in St. Louis, MO. Mr. Greeley is a member of the faculties of The Estes Park Institute, the American College of Physician Executives, and The Medical Leadership Forum of the Governance Institute.

Mr. Greeley has held a number of positions with the JCAHO. A founding member of InterQual, he served as vice president for professional services at Kenosha (WI) Hospital and Medical Center. Mr. Greeley's career spans nearly 20 years, during which time he has conducted more than 2,000 seminars on subjects relating to credentialing, governance responsibilities, antitrust, and other health care-related subjects.

Jay Coburn is the vice president and managing director of The Greeley Company, a firm specializing in providing consulting and educational services to health care leaders. An experienced hospital systems designer and implementer, he has held administrative positions at Massachusetts General Hospital and Elliot Hospital (Manchester, NH), and was previously a senior consulting manager with Arthur Andersen & Co. Mr. Coburn writes, speaks, and regularly consults on leadership, managed care readiness, quality improvement, and health care accreditation topics.

Table of Contents

Preface

The Joint Commission on Accreditation of Healthcare Organizations (JCAHO) is now recognizing what we've known all along—the information that a hospital collects and uses is invaluable to its success. By bringing together the many standards governing patient records, data processing, information integrity and security, and library resources, the JCAHO is forcing a rare alliance in hospitals—having departments work and depend on one another. This alliance, based on the need for communication across many areas of the hospital, is vitally important to meeting the information management standards and to the survey process as a whole.

Effective information management will play a critical role in a hospital's response to the transformation of the information delivery system. After all, a hospital cannot function without the proper management of information or communication—the care of every patient and the work of all staff depend on it. Therefore, the standards, and in particular the information management standards, will require teamwork on the part of everyone who manages any kind of information in the hospital.

Forming and maintaining this alliance across departments poses new challenges and exciting new avenues for improvement. The information management standards provide a genuine opportunity for those of us who have been touting the importance of information management. No longer will information management be the job of a few—now, most departments and areas are required to have some sort of information management plan. The JCAHO has elevated information management to a hospital-wide activity, emphasizing the importance and necessity of information in the hospital. This gives us the opportunity to use our knowledge of information processes and transfer it to others, fostering teamwork and cooperation.

Take IM.6, integration and retention, for example; this standard talks about bringing information together from various systems. It underscores that information management is not an island activity, but one in which health care information must cross departmental and even organizational lines to be of optimal use.

We've known about the gold mine that exists in clinical databases, detailed medical records, computerized reports, and library references. Now, the JCAHO acknowledges the critical usefulness of having such data available, understood, and used. Not only does the information gathered in the hospital play a vital role in patient care, it may also reveal numerous areas for improving organization-wide processes. By tapping into the different types of information available in a hospital, a hospital can plan to integrate information processes throughout its organization.

The standards also encourage an information management process that exhibits successful stages of planning, controlling, analyzing, and improving. By requiring practical and succinct information management processes, the JCAHO has moved beyond mere policies and procedures and has developed a concept based on accuracy and performance.

Yet the information management standards—for all the good they propose—bring challenges, opportunities, and even confusion. Because of these obstacles, there exists the need for interpretation, clarification, and a method to make them fall into place in a reasonable manner and timetable that is consistent with a hospital's overall goals and capabilities. That's where this book can help. We applaud the publication of *Information Management—The Compliance Guide to the JCAHO Standards*. It is a publication that explains the standards, analyzes what JCAHO surveyors will review, and most importantly, outlines a team approach to managing information. We know you will find this book a valuable tool to help your hospital comply with the information management standards.

John Glaser, PhD
Vice President, Information Systems
Brigham and Women's Hospital

Jill Fainter
Assistant Vice President
Columbia HCA Healthcare Corp.

John Glaser, PhD, is vice president of information systems at Brigham and Women's Hospital in Boston, Massachusetts. He was chairman and is currently on the board of trustees of the College of Healthcare Information Management Executives. Dr. Glaser is a faculty member and lecturer at many institutions, including the Harvard School of Public Health and the University of Michigan. He has published numerous articles on the subject of information management.

Jill Fainter is assistant vice president for quality assurance support at the corporate offices of Columbia HCA Healthcare Corporation in Nashville, Tennessee. She was a director on the board of the American Health Information Management Association and is a member of the JCAHO's Professional and Technical Advisory Committee. Additionally, she served on the JCAHO task force that developed the 1994 Management of Information (IM) standards.

Chapter 1
Introduction

Chapter 1
Introduction

Your institution must deal with enormous volumes of data. It uses, abuses, devours, and generates data—sometimes turning it into useful information—information that, like it or not, is an integral and important part of your institution's delivery of care.

The Joint Commission on Accreditation of Healthcare Organizations (JCAHO) has long been concerned with the quality and accessibility of patient information in the patient record. And, recent years have seen it call for an increase in the use of information in monitoring quality.

The JCAHO's Agenda for Change brought with it a great leap forward, with interest in and surveyor involvement with virtually every aspect of information generation and use in hospitals. A chapter of the *Comprehensive Accreditation Manual for Hospitals (CAMH)* is devoted to information management, which emphasizes effective organization-wide information management. This creates challenges for many individuals, for example:

- ◆ Information managers have to be actively involved in a JCAHO survey.

- ◆ Medical records managers have to address the analysis and use of aggregate patient information.

- ◆ Quality managers have to consider the information management standards because they directly relate to the requirements for performance improvement.

- ◆ Hospital leaders are faced with developing and implementing an information plan and integrating it with the other mandated organization-wide plans.

- ◆ Survey coordinators must be prepared for a multidisciplinary review of the hospital.

The real world ——————————————————————————————

JCAHO standards for information management and what will constitute compliance will be the topic of discussion in hospitals all over the country. And in order to comply, you may not wish to rely on the somewhat artificial outline of the standards. Instead, your time and effort should be allocated to organizing the important aspects of information planning. Your institution will want to focus on activities that will both produce real benefits and comply with JCAHO requirements.

With this in mind, we think you will find this book unique. Two major projects have been designed to cover information planning and patient records. Tasks, responsibilities, work plans, checklists, and sample reports are provided to help you organize and tailor a practical and workable multi-department effort.

The results of these two projects will be valuable on their own merits. We're confident that surveyors will observe that your institution has gone a long way toward complying with the letter and the spirit of the new standards.

How to use this book ——————————————————————————

Information Management—The Compliance Guide to the JCAHO Standards will assist you in planning your hospital's information management (IM) agenda with material found in the following chapters.

Start by reading **Chapter 2**. It is a summary of the JCAHO's 1998 IM standards and includes elements of what will constitute compliance, an analysis of what surveyors may look for during survey, and required documents for review. This is a summary, not a detailed explanation of the IM standards. If you have not already done so, secure a copy of the *CAMH* and its corresponding scoring guidelines and read the Management of Information (IM) chapter. It is essential that you become familiar with the standards and scoring guidelines as it will be easier for you to follow the ideas, projects, and activities provided in this book. Also read the introduction to the *CAMH* to see why the JCAHO views IM as integral to accreditation. You should note that the JCAHO recently lifted all of its scoring caps on the IM standards and all standards will be scored on a scale of 1–5.

Begin the project in **Chapter 3**. This chapter discusses an information planning project covering the preparation and organization of all information in the hospital. It focuses on assessing needs and opportunities for improvement, identifying priorities, and defining management strategies and policies, all of which lead to the final development of an information management plan. It calls for the establishment of a project team and emphasizes the importance of the organization's support. **Chapter 3** will be of significant, ongoing value to those people in your organization who rely on timely and accurate information.

Read **Chapter 4** and get this project underway, regardless of how close you are to your next survey. This chapter describes how to make sure patient records are in compliance with IM.7 and other patient-records related standards. It identifies areas for performance improvement and provides examples, forms, and charts to facilitate preparation. Key providers, users of patient information, and the quality manager should be included in this project.

Finally, no matter when your next survey is scheduled, read **Chapter 5**. It outlines how to prepare for the document review session and other IM-related interviews that will take place during the survey.

Chapter 2
The IM Standards

Chapter 2
The IM Standards

This chapter covers the JCAHO survey process for those sessions that focus on information management, including the document review session, the information management interview, and the medical records interview. A summary of each IM standard (IM.1–IM.10) is included with specific requirements of each standard, an explanation of the standard's intent, pointers on how the standard may be surveyed, and a list of the documents that should be provided to show compliance.

The survey process

The chapter on the Management of Information (IM) contains many standards that affect a broad cross-section of the hospital. This means that all departments will be expected to have knowledge of information management, including the medical staff. Surveyors will look for compliance and an understanding of the IM standards.

The document review session
The JCAHO has shifted its survey emphasis away from written department policies and procedures and toward more interviews and observations. But, there remain important requirements for documents that are complete and well organized.

The document review session on the first day of survey sets the stage for the rest of the survey by influencing and directing surveyor comments, observations, and questions. One focus of this session, held without hospital participation, is on documentation that shows compliance with the IM standards. For example, surveyors will want to see the past year's medical record reviews.

The information management interview
The second day of survey will include the information management interview. Its purpose is to assess the hospital's information planning processes and approaches. The attendees may include the Chief

Information Officer (CIO), information services director, medical records director, resource center director or librarian, as well as other key people involved with information management. The interview will be conducted by the administrative surveyor and will address specific IM standards. IM-specific documentation is reviewed in the document review session.

This interview session will focus on the main issues outlined in the standards: the hospital's information management system (plan and implementation), confidentiality, the definition and internal and external use of data, and the accessibility of information throughout the hospital.

During this interview, the surveyor will ask pointed questions related to the IM standards. Some of these questions may be based on observations from the document review session or patient unit visits. The sections in this chapter on how the standards may be surveyed include a sample of areas surveyors may cover. Use these sections to prepare individuals who will be asked to attend the IM interview.

The medical record review
This survey activity is twofold—hospitals are required to complete medical record information for the medical record interview and review closed records against a tally sheet in that interview. Results and information management issues will also be discussed in the interview. These survey sessions are intended to address all standards for which the source of data is the medical record. The review will include most of IM.7, which covers the requirements for patient-specific information.

A sample of about 20 records will be requested by the surveyor, based on the hospital's size and surveyor observations from the document review session. The list of records for review will be given to the hospital after the document review session. The hospital is expected to gather the requested records and complete a form called Medical Records Statistics, which deals with record delinquency and the history and physical and operative report in the record for the past 12 months. This form should be included with the closed records and brought to the medical records interview.

The medical record review will be performed by medical records staff during the medical record interview. Each participant will be given a JCAHO medical record tally sheet to use to compare the records against specific documentation standards. The results of the review are tallied for surveyor review to determine compliance. (See Chapter 5 for more information.)

The documentation improvement project in Chapter 4 will help prepare your hospital for the medical record review.

Review of the standards —————————————————————————

IM.1 Information management planning

Explanation

IM.1 and its related standards require hospitals to plan and design their information management systems around the needs of the organization. These standards emphasize the availability of support for various activities as well as continuous performance improvement. Organizations must also consider information systems that are appropriate for their size and complexity as well as provide the proper staff, services, and systems to support them.

The JCAHO lists in the intent the following factors that it expects hospitals to assess when planning to meet future information needs:
- the organization's type, structure, and complexity;
- the needs of individuals/groups whom the function serves or will serve (for example, governance, leaders, clinical staff, inpatients and ambulatory patients, patients' families, payers, purchasers, regulatory bodies, accrediting bodies), and support needed for planning purposes;
- the data and support needed for education services and any research activity;
- any national and state guidelines for data set parity and connectivity in interfacing information systems;
- the requirements for internal and external transmission of information;
- longitudinal information reporting needs;
- the data and information to support continuous performance improvement;
- the requirements for comparing the organization's performance with internal past performance, other organizations' performance, and with information from literature, for example, on practice guidelines or benchmarking;

- the appropriateness of various technologies;
- the costs of various technologies;
- the need to support customer and supplier relationships;
- analysis of resource use for patients with particular clinical problems to enhance the cost-effectiveness of care;
- the enhancement of work flow activity;
- the support needed for administrative and clinical decision-making;
- the direction needed to look at the complexity of services provided; for example, library services, medical records, and computer services;
- long-range plans that affect information needs; and
- needs based on the organization's mission, goals, services, staff, mode of delivery, resources, and access to technology.

Compliance with IM.1 will be a lengthy process for most hospitals. There-fore, even though the standards and the scoring guidelines do not require a written plan, hospitals would be wise to develop one. According to the standards, an effective plan requires input and continuous support from the entire organization.

Specifics of the standard

- ◆ IM.1.1 states all information-management processes be appropriate for the size and complexity of services.
- ◆ IM.1.1.1 mandates management, staffing, and resources be appropriate.
- ◆ IM.1.1.2 insists that the assessment of information needs be multidisciplinary.

Intent

The JCAHO's intent in these standards is to make sure all organizations assess their needs based on an analysis of internal and external needs. This analysis should provide the organization with data on what all areas of the organization need for information, as well as outside services, companies, and agencies. Patient care, research, education, and management decisions all depend on the activities related to this standard.

How the standard may be surveyed

This standard may be surveyed in two principal areas:

- ◆ the leadership interview and
- ◆ the information management interview.

The leadership interview may focus on:
- ◆ your hospital's information management systems and
- ◆ how they meet the needs of the organization.

The information management interview may focus on:
- ◆ your hospital's planning process for managing patient and aggregate clinical data,
- ◆ the information staff use in their decision-making, and
- ◆ who is responsible for information systems.

Documents to be provided
- ◆ Minutes, reports, and other documentation that show evidence that the hospital assessed its information needs and planned accordingly to meet them.

IM.2 Care of information

Explanation
IM.2 requires that all clinical information—including medical records—is confidential, secure, complete, and safe from physical damage. The intent says hospitals should:
- identify the individuals who may access information;
- identify the information each may access;
- have a policy for an individual's confidentiality obligation;
- state when the release of information and removal of records is authorized, i.e., court order, subpoena, or statute; and
- define the process to be followed when confidentiality and security are breached.

Specifics of the standard
Only the accompanying standards—IM.2.1, IM.2.2, and IM.2.3—are scored. These standards pertain to different aspects of the care of information.

Levels of security—IM.2.1 requires hospitals to determine the need for different levels of security for different types of information. To score a 1 on this standard, the hospital must have both a process and a plan in place.

Easy retrieval of information—IM.2.2 expects hospitals to retrieve all kinds of information easily without compromising security.

Sensitive information—IM.2.3 requires the hospital to protect information that's especially sensitive. The hospital must have a security mechanism and enforce it to safeguard records or information against unauthorized access or tampering.

Removing records—The intent says the hospital must have a policy stating that it takes a court order, subpoena, or statute to remove records from the hospital's jurisdiction.

Intent

The JCAHO's intent in these standards is for the organization to take on the responsibility of protecting its information, which includes who has access, the extent of access, maintenance of confidentiality, and the release and security of information.

How the standard may be surveyed

The standard may be surveyed in two principal areas:
- ◆ the information management interview and
- ◆ the medical record interview.

The information management interview may focus on the system that monitors confidentiality, security, and the integrity of patient records.

The medical record interview may include discussion on:
- ◆ 24-hour accessibility of records and
- ◆ identifying the policies and procedures that reflect that accessibility.

Documents to be provided

- ◆ Policies on appropriate levels of security and confidentiality for information and data.
- ◆ Hospital-wide and medical staff policies pertaining to the removal of patient records.
- ◆ Evidence that the confidentiality of patient-specific information and privacy for sensitive records is maintained.
- ◆ Evidence showing the hospital safeguards records from damage, loss, or tampering.

IM.3 Capture of data

Explanation
The IM.3 standards focus on getting hospitals to standardize the methods by which they use and distribute information. It requires that a uniform method for data capture be in place. The hospital should use and reference any external or industry standards that will make data comparisons possible with other hospitals. It is important that data collection be accurate, timely, and cost-efficient.

Hospitals must also demonstrate that they look for the presence, accuracy, and timeliness of 19 specific items in the medical record. These standards require hospitals to review the medical records completion on an ongoing basis. The medical staff, along with other hospital staff as appropriate, must perform the review. The review must include each record or a representative sample of records.

Specifics of the standard
- IM.3.1 insists that hospitals standardize data sets, definitions, codes, classifications, and terms used throughout the hospital.
- IM.3.2 calls for the timely, efficient, and accurate collection of data.
- The intent statement expects hospitals to ensure that
    - abbreviations and symbols are standardized;
    - data are unbiased and accurate;
    - a quality control system is in place; and
    - standardization complies with state and federal regulations.
- IM.3.2.1 states hospitals must review the completeness, accuracy, and timely completion of medical records on an ongoing basis and show that action was taken to improve the process.
- IM.3.2.1.1 says a representative sample of records should be included in the review.
- The intent says the medical records review must
    - look at the completion and timeliness of 19 specific items in the medical record,
    - review a department's scope of practice,
    - include inpatient records, and
    - review annually the records of each physician on the medical staff.

Intent

The JCAHO intends these standards to facilitate an organization's comparability within itself and among other facilities. The fact that the hospital is working toward this particular system of data capture and review should be clearly outlined or documented. IM.3 has important references to medical record review, making sure that accuracy, timeliness, and authentication of data are addressed and the hospital looks at delinquent records.

How the standard may be surveyed

The standard may be surveyed in three principal areas:
- ◆ the information management interview,
- ◆ the medical record interview, and
- ◆ during patient unit visits.

The information management interview and review of records may focus on your hospital's uniform data definitions and capture methods.

The content and clinical pertinence of the medical record may be discussed and reviewed during the medical record interview and patient unit visits. This may include documentation of donated and received transplants and autopsy results.

Documents to be provided
- ◆ Policies and procedures that reflect medical records content for accuracy, timely completion, completeness and clinical pertinence.
- ◆ Minutes or reports from the group that reviews medical records outlining quality of documentation and timely completion for the most recent 12 months.

IM.4 Information management education

Explanation

IM.4 requires that the key people who generate, collect, and analyze data and who make information-related decisions be educated on the principles of information management. Education should include
- security and confidentiality issues,
- measurement techniques and quality tools to make data into useable information,

- data collection training,
- data interpretation,
- how to use data in decision-making,
- patient and family education processes for care, and
- development of indicators to improve processes.

Organizations must prove that staff are educated according to their individual needs and responsibilities.

Intent
The JCAHO's intent of this standard is to make sure hospitals educate staff members who participate in information management.

How the standard may be surveyed
IM.4 will likely be surveyed through face-to-face interviews between surveyors and staff throughout the hospital.

Department directors and managers may have to describe the type of information management education they received.

Documents to be provided
◆ Education outlines, assessed needs, objectives, agendas, and evaluation criteria that pertain to individual information management needs.
◆ Evidence that supports staff participation in information management education.

IM.5 Transmission of information

Explanation
IM.5 promotes the timely and accurate transmission of data and stresses a standardized format. Examples include the pharmacy avoiding abbreviations and medical records being accessible 24 hours a day. It is important to balance timeliness with policies on safeguarding information (IM.2). IM.5.1 says data transmission formats and methods must be standardized.

Intent
IM.5 is intended to ensure that hospitals effectively communicate data and transmit it on time, do so in an accurate manner, and retain the data's

integrity. The standards also emphasize that information be available in a time frame to support important decisions.

How the standard may be surveyed

This standard may be surveyed in three principal areas:

- ◆ during medical staff and nursing leadership interviews,
- ◆ the medical record interview, and
- ◆ the information management interview.

Medical staff and nursing leadership interviews may focus on:

- ◆ the format and organization of the medical record to determine if it is designed to accommodate the needs of all users;
- ◆ the hospital's policies for patient records being available at all times; and
- ◆ orders being acted on and diagnostic test results being available in a timely manner.

The medical record interview may include discussion on medical records being available 24 hours a day and the policies or systems related to that requirement.

The information management interview may cover the standardization of transmission formats and methods and if they meet the users' needs.

Documents to be provided

- ◆ None specific to this standard.

IM.6 Integration and retention

Explanation

IM.6 concerns data requirements for linkage, reporting, and retention. Hospitals must show that patient and nonpatient data is coordinated; can be linked, organized, analyzed, and interpreted; and provides longitudinal information. For example, there should be linkages to support patient care and hospital management, internal and external information, and information from clinical and nonclinical literature. This standard also requires medical records be retained based on legal regulations and usage patterns for patient care, research, and educational needs.

Intent

IM.6 focuses on the integration of information systems, making sure that all systems are compatible and information can be gathered from every other system in the organization. This linkage concerns both internal and external systems that relate to the improvement of patient care. IM.6.1 spotlights the importance of retaining medical records for legal and other reasons and the enforcement of this policy throughout the hospital.

How the standard may be surveyed

This standard may be surveyed in six principal areas:
- the information management interview,
- the pharmacy visit,
- the performance improvement interview,
- department director interviews, and
- patient unit visits.

The information management interview may address the systems in place that integrate information throughout the hospital.

Surveyors may look for the location of authorized DEA numbers in the pharmacy department.

The performance improvement interview may focus on evidence of how the hospital links data for patient care and organizational functions.

During department director interviews and patient unit visits, surveyors may ask how the organization makes current literature available.

Documents to be provided
- Policies that state the length of time records are kept.

IM.7 Patient-specific information

Explanation

IM.7 is the longest section of the IM chapter because it deals with the content requirements for medical records. There are nine main topics to this section of standards.

Specifics of the standard

Authority of individuals—IM.7.1 emphasizes that any patient treated in any setting must have a medical record. IM.7.1.1 states that any person who documents patient care-related information in medical records must be authorized to do so by hospital and medical staff policy.

Record content—IM.7.2 says the hospital must ensure the medical record has proper patient information. The intent includes 26 items every medical record must contain:

- each patient's name, address, date of birth, and the name of any legally authorized representative;
- legal status for patients receiving mental health services;
- any emergency care provided to the patient prior to arrival;
- the record and findings of the patient's assessment;
- conclusions or impressions drawn from the medical history and physical examination;
- diagnosis or diagnostic impression;
- reason(s) for admission or treatment;
- goals of treatment and the treatment plan;
- evidence of known advance directives;
- evidence of informed consent required by organizational policy;
- any diagnosis and therapeutic orders;
- all diagnostic and therapeutic procedures and tests performed and the results;
- all operative and other invasive procedures performed, using acceptable disease and operative terminology that includes etiology, as appropriate;
- progress notes made by the medical staff and other authorized individuals;
- all reassessments or revisions of the treatment plan, when necessary;
- clinical observations;
- response to the care provided;
- consultation reports;
- every medication ordered or prescribed for an inpatient;
- each medication dispensed to or prescribed for an ambulatory patient or an inpatient on discharge;
- every dose of medication administered and any adverse drug reactions;
- all relevant diagnoses established during the course of care;

◆ any referrals or communications made to external or internal
care providers and to community agencies;
◆ conclusions at termination of hospitalization;
◆ discharge instructions of patient and family; and
◆ clinical resumes, discharge summaries, final progress note, or
transfer summary.

The intent is specific about the clinical resume, saying that on discharge the
resume contains all relevant and important information for continuous care.

The intent also goes on to specify that patients with minor problems (as
defined by the medical staff) can have a progress note substitute for the
clinical resume if hospitalization is less than 48 hours. The intent allows for
a transfer summary if patients are moved to different levels of care within
the organization.

Surgical documentation—IM.7.3 addresses the documentation of surgical
care, including anesthesia. IM.7.3.1 and IM.7.3.2 mention that reports of
surgical procedures must include the practitioner responsible for the
surgery, be completed immediately after surgery, and contain the findings,
procedures used, specimen removed, postoperative diagnosis, and names
of the primary surgeon and assistants.

IM.7.3.2.1 states that the surgeon must authenticate the report as soon as
possible. If there is a technical delay, such as for transcription, IM.7.3.2.2
says the surgeon must provide an operative progress note as soon as possible after surgery.

IM.7.3.3 covers the components of appropriate postoperative documentation. IM.7.3.4 and IM.7.3.4.1 state that postoperative documentation records
the discharge of a patient from the recovery area made by a licensed independent practitioner and that the discharge is based on discharge criteria
approved by the medical staff.

Ambulatory records—Standards IM.7.4 and IM.7.4.1 state that the records of
patients receiving ambulatory services must contain a list of diagnoses,
conditions, procedures, allergies, adverse reactions, and medications. A list
of these items should be kept for those ambulatory patients who receive
ongoing treatment (three or more times in a six-month period).

Emergency records—IM.7.5 and IM.7.5.1 require additional information to be included in emergency records, such as the time and means of arrival, conclusions, and documentation if the patient leaves against medical advice.

IM.7.5.2 addresses the discharge of an emergency patient, stating the medical record must include care notes, disposition, condition, and follow-up instructions. Patient authorization to release information for follow-up care to his or her physician or health care organization is addressed in IM.7.5.3.

Records completion—IM.7.6 addresses the timeliness of the completion of medical records. Record completion for discharged patients must not exceed 30 days. The intent includes detailed information on important measurements for delinquent records completion. The hospital must measure delinquency at least every three months and report the findings as part of the medical record review in order to be in compliance.

Verbal orders—IM.7.7 dictates that verbal orders must be accepted and transcribed by qualified personnel. The intent says that hospitals may decide when, how, and if verbal orders are authenticated, and the JCAHO only requires you to authenticate an order if a state or federal law or regulation or hospital policy requires it.

Authentication—IM.7.8 addresses the authentication of entries in the medical record. The JCAHO requires hospitals to date and identify the author of every medical record, but it no longer requires hospitals to authenticate each and every entry. Now, your hospital may decide for itself which entries it feels must be authenticated, with the exception of entries for histories, physical exams, operative procedures, consultations, and discharge summaries, which the JCAHO still requires every hospital to authenticate.

Unified record—IM.7.9 says that hospitals must be able to assemble and have accessible all relevent information from a patient's record when the patient is admitted or seen for ambulatory or emergency care.

Intent

The patient record is the most critical information resource in the hospital for patient care delivery. For this reason, the JCAHO has placed added emphasis on these standards to ensure quality. The medical record is also used as principal evidence of the patient care process.

How the standard may be surveyed
This standard may be surveyed in two principal areas:
- ◆ the medical record review and
- ◆ during patient unit visits.

The medical record interview will focus on:
- ◆ the timely completion of medical records;
- ◆ histories and physicals, medical office history and physical completion within 30 days, readmission history and assessment, and autopsy result timeliness;
- ◆ evidence of advance directives;
- ◆ evidence of informed consent;
- ◆ verbal orders;
- ◆ dated entries;
- ◆ physician authentication;
- ◆ operative and other invasive procedure notations;
- ◆ progress notes;
- ◆ reporting of autopsy results;
- ◆ prescribed medication upon discharge;
- ◆ operative reports written or dictated after surgery, authenticated, and operative progress noted immediately after surgery;
- ◆ operative report includes findings, procedures, specimens removed, postoperative diagnosis, and the name of the surgeon/assistant;
- ◆ for ambulatory patients: list of diagnoses, medications, conditions, allergies, and procedures by third visit; and
- ◆ for emergency care patients: final disposition, condition, and instructions for care at termination of treatment.

Patient unit visits may focus on:
- ◆ clinical pertinence of the medical record;
- ◆ the assembly of records for patients who receive emergency, inpatient, or ambulatory care; and
- ◆ caregiver knowledge of medical record content.

Documents to be provided

- ◆ All related policies on medical record content.
- ◆ Policies and procedures on treatments or procedures that need informed consent documentation.
- ◆ Policies and procedures related to the recording of operative reports.
- ◆ Policies and procedures on the content and timely completion of medical records.
- ◆ Rules and regulations pertaining to medical staff verbal orders for medication and who authenticates them.
- ◆ Policies and procedures on the methods to authenticate entries into the medical record.
- ◆ A summary or written description of the system that assembles all inpatient, emergency, and ambulatory records for scheduled and non-scheduled patient care, when required.

IM.8 Aggregate information

Explanation

IM.8 requires hospitals to collect and analyze aggregate data to support decision-making, operations, performance improvement activities, and patient care. It calls for data to be defined, captured, analyzed, transmitted, compared, and reported with the ultimate goal of their being aggregated to support managerial and organizational functions, and used to improve processes.

Specifics of the standard

- ◆ The intent of the standard requires hospitals to aggregate data for the following:
  - the pharmacy to control and account for all drugs as required by law;
  - discuss information related to hazards and safety practices, including failures or errors in safety-related areas (equipment management, utilities management), documented semiannual surveys that address environmental hazards and unsafe practices, and documentation on property damage or occupational injuries;
  - radionuclides and radiopharmaceutical records have the radionuclide identity, date received, method of receipt, activity, recipient's name, date administered, and disposal;
  - records of any required reporting to proper authorities;

- diagnoses and performed procedures;
- patient demographic information
- financial information;
- measuring performance improvement and documenting organization-wide activities;
- aggregate data to be collected on licensed independent practitioners for use in performance improvement activities, decision-making, and patient care;
- the organization to gather accurate, timely information for decision-making and planning purposes; and
- the organization gathers data to support clinical research.

♦ Coding and retrieval systems aggregate data by
- diagnosis and procedure,
- patient demographic information, and
- financial information.

♦ The control register for emergency and outpatient services to have particular patient information, including
- name, age, and gender;
- date, time, and means of arrival;
- complaint;
- disposition; and
- departure time.

Intent

Clinical and administrative data are to be aggregated to support managerial decisions, track trends, make comparisons internally and externally, and improve performance. The JCAHO wants leaders to use aggregate information as a prerequisite to assessing opportunities and evaluating results.

How the standard may be surveyed

This standard may be surveyed in 14 principal areas:
♦ the leadership interview
♦ medical staff and nursing leadership interviews,
♦ information management interview,
♦ CEO interview,
♦ plant, technology, and safety management,
♦ the resource center,

- ◆ strategic planning and resource allocation interview,
- ◆ emergency services visits,
- ◆ ambulatory unit visits,
- ◆ the pharmacy visit,
- ◆ department director interviews,
- ◆ patient unit visits, and
- ◆ in the review of medical staff credentials files.

Leaders from the above areas, including the CEO, department directors, and those selected for the information management interview, may be called on to identify the aggregate data used to support their decisions for patient care, department activities, assessments, and performance improvement.

The medical staff and nursing leadership interviews may focus on determining if the system that gathers practitioner-specific data is adequate.

The information management interview may focus on the coding and retrieval system as well as unusual events or complications.

Review of plant, technology, and safety management may focus on:
- ◆ how the department collects information on safety hazards and practices;
- ◆ how that data is used to identify safety management issues; and
- ◆ what types of aggregate data are used.

Resource center staff should be able to explain the types of aggregate data available to department directors for decision-making and performance improvement activities.

Surveyors in the strategic planning and resource allocation interview may look for the coding and retrieval systems used for financial data.

During the emergency services and ambulatory unit visits, staff may be asked to explain the control register process.

In the pharmacy, surveyors may ask how physicians' signatures are verified when prescribing medication.

All staff identified during patient unit visits should be able to explain the types of aggregate data available for decision-making, operations, and performance improvement activities.

In the review of medical staff credentials files, data should be available that describes how the performance of licensed independent practitioners is assessed.

In addition, surveyors will focus on the systems that track performance improvement–related data in most areas.

Documents to be provided
- ◆ Any documentation that relates to the assessment of needs for the use of aggregate information.
- ◆ Optional: A list of regular and ad hoc reports available to hospital and medical staff leaders.

IM.9 Knowledge-based information

Explanation
IM.9 focuses on the management of knowledge-based information, making sure appropriate resources are available for staff use in education, research, analysis, managerial decisions, and improving processes. Knowledge-based information must have proper resources and services to assist professional staff, support decision-making, support performance improvement, meet research needs, and educate patients and families.

IM.9.1 says knowledge-based information must be up to date, authoritative, and available to staff and patients. Resources include databases, publications, audiovisual materials, and electronic information. The intent of this standard also says resources must be provided efficiently and promptly, and poison control and formulary information are available when needed.

IM.9.2 says hospitals must assess the needs of certain groups, including the medical and nursing staffs, administrators, other hospital staff, students, patients and their families, and researchers. The needs assessment should address accessibility, timeliness, and the internal and external linkage of information. The intent says library services must respond to requests, anticipate information needs, link literature to the hospital's processes, and provide current, accurate information based on needs. The standards also address the location of information, saying information should be accessible at the work site, in a library, and from outside sources. Service quality will be judged by the accuracy of the information, currency, relevance, speed of response, ease of use, and validity.

Intent

These standards focus on helping hospital staff, especially those in professional roles, gather knowledge and maintain their skills to improve patient care and support their decisions. This standard suggests hospitals assess knowledge-based information needs, accessibility, and systems. This standard does not require hospital libraries to possess all needed resources. Sharing arrangements can be arranged, which should provide timely access to literature and other resources not available on-site.

How the standard may be surveyed

This standard may be surveyed in six principal areas:
- ◆ medical and nursing staff interviews,
- ◆ the pharmacy visit,
- ◆ the resource center visit,
- ◆ department director interviews,
- ◆ patient unit visits, and
- ◆ the strategic planning and resource allocation interview.

Medical and nursing staff interviews may focus on access to knowledge-based information specific to patient care, clinical activities, and research.

The pharmacy and patient unit visits may focus on:
- ◆ immediate access to poison control information and resources and
- ◆ the availability of the hospital formulary to users.

The resource center visit, department director interviews, and patient unit visits may focus on:
- ◆ resource center information that is currently available to hospital staff,
- ◆ how the system works,
- ◆ who is responsible for the availability of the information, and
- ◆ policies specific to the availability of this information.

During the resource center visit, the surveyor may ask about the assessment processes for knowledge-based information needs, with emphasis on timeliness, accessibility, and linkage to internal systems and external databases.

The strategic planning and resource allocation interview may focus on:
- the resources available to staff and
- if they meet the needs of the organization.

Documents to be provided
- Surveys, minutes, reports, or plans that demonstrate evidence that the hospital has assessed its needs for knowledge-based information.

IM.10 Comparative data

Explanation
IM.10 says comparative performance data must be defined, collected, analyzed, reported, and used consistently with state and federal guidelines. The other standards require hospitals to use external databases (IM.10.1), contribute to external databases (IM.10.2), and maintain confidentiality and security when contributing (IM.10.3).

Intent
The JCAHO says the intent of this standard is to "develop [the hospital's] future capabilities and goals." This means that hospitals should use external databases and internal data to compare performance and identify trends, and contribute data to other organizations. Hospitals should also set their own benchmarks by collecting data internally and comparing past performance.

How the standard will be surveyed
This standard may be surveyed in three principal areas:
- the medical staff and nursing leadership interviews,
- information management interview, and
- the medical record review.

The above areas may include discussions on:
- the types of external databases used and
- how data is used for comparison.

Documents to be provided

◆ A list of the external comparative databases used by the hospital with a description of how that information is used in performance improvement activities.

Chapter 3

The Information Management Project

Chapter 3
The Information Management Project

We live in the information age and are constantly faced with the challenge of turning mountains of raw data into usable information. Although technology can help with that challenge, it presents problems; namely, how to manage, control, and utilize new information that can change with unbelievable rapidity. What was state-of-the-art technology last year is now available, affordable, and should be included in your information tool kit.

Even if you recently completed an information plan, or follow the activities described in this chapter, the job of planning is never done. You and your institution will need to revisit the questions of strategy, control, quality, use, and organization of information on a regular basis.

There are three objectives for this chapter:
- ◆ Describe an information project made up of five major activities:

    - Define a baseline for current information capabilities
    - Identify future needs and uses for information
    - Develop strategies to satisfy those needs
    - Establish information management policies
    - Set priorities and create a plan to accomplish your institution's information goals
    (See figure 3.1 for a visual representation of the project.)

- ◆ Offer a range of involvement for information management-related activities that will apply to hospitals with different capabilities and resources.

- ◆ Cross-reference the activities, where applicable, to the JCAHO's IM standards.

Figure 3.1

The Information Management Project

Define a baseline

Get help → Identify customers → Take inventory → Confirm budget → Establish ground rules

Identify future needs

Consider opportunities for improvement → Identify information needs not met → Develop project descriptions

Develop strategies

Patient record → Integration → Emergency preparedness → Information systems and technology → Library services

Establish information management policies

Important organization IM policies

Set priorities and create a plan

Estimate time and resources → Review priorities of projects → Draft implementation plan

Define an information baseline —————————————

Five major activities will get the information management project underway in an organized and realistic fashion by first defining an information baseline. The five activities are as follows:

1. Get help and involve the organization,

2. Identify current information customers,

3. Take an inventory of current information capabilities,

4. Confirm the information budget and organization constraints, and

5. Establish ground rules for prioritizing projects.

For each of these activities, two points of reference will be offered: *At a minimum* will describe the level of involvement achievable for smaller hospitals, which may have limited time and resources; *If time permits* will expand the activities for larger institutions.

1. Get help and involve the organization

At a minimum
A working group, a decision group, and a facilitator should be involved from start to finish.

A working group is needed to contribute detailed facts and ideas and to conduct most of the activities in this chapter. It will answer questions, provide input, and make sure the project is grounded in reality. Its members should be people who are most involved with developing and using information. The working group may be composed of the administrative staff or a selection of department heads. Generally, a group of five or six is manageable.

A decision group will not only make the major decisions concerning future information strategies, projects, and policies, but will also be responsible for communicating the results of the information project, on a formal basis, to the governing board and the medical staff. The decision group should be composed of the CEO, the chief nurse executive, and representatives from the governing board and the medical staff. This makeup will help satisfy several JCAHO standards and will go a long way toward turning the project's results into actions.

A facilitator is needed to take responsibility for the project. This individual will set agendas, unite the working and decision groups, compile information, and document results. Candidates for the position may include data processing managers, medical records managers, or any other manager with significant interest in information management and a willingness to take on added work. One important point should not be ignored: This project, even at a minimum, will take time. The facilitator will need an allowance of one or two days a week for the information project's responsibilities.

If time permits
A full-time project leader should be assigned to the information project. He or she can easily stay busy with activities and will assist in moving the project toward completion. Advisory groups can also provide input during the planning process and provide support when projects are implemented. Additional groups can be created for further detailed information and analysis, if needed.

Regardless of the number of advisors or groups, a decision group is vital to the success of the project. Its support and involvement will be crucial to harnessing the energy of the organization behind the information project.

The above activity addresses IM.1, which stipulates appropriate support for planning purposes, in research activities, and for decision-making.

2. Identify current information customers

At a minimum
Develop a list of current information providers and users (internal and external customers) and pass it through the decision group for review and approval. This list will help in creating a complete inventory of current information capabilities and uses. Hospital staff who are named on the list should receive a questionnaire on their information capabilities (see the next activity for details). The facilitator, a member of the working group, or an interested manager should research the capabilities of data for external users.

If time permits

Consider future information strategies by adding *potential* information providers and users to the customer list. This may assist the working and decision groups in deciding what projects to consider for implementation, especially if improvements to a system will help potential users. No user or group should be ruled out due to budget constraints or conflicting priorities. The decision group can determine which groups or users should be included, based on its understanding of the hospital's overall strategic plan. Any documentation generated from this step should be reviewed and approved by the decision group and retained for future JCAHO scrutiny.

The above activity addresses IM.1 by assessing the users or groups the facility serves or who provide information services. It also identifies the need to support customer relationships.

3. Take an inventory of current information capabilities

At a minimum

The working group and the facilitator should compile an inventory of the hospital's current information capabilities. All internal information users and providers (identified in the last step) should complete an inventory questionnaire. The questionnaire should ask about the following topics:
- automated systems' use and adequacy,
- databases generated and used by each system,
- data elements in each database,
- standard reports,
- interfaces where information is moved between systems,
- reports provided to external organizations,
- system strengths,
- system weaknesses, and
- desired improvements.

When the questionnaires are completed, the facilitator should follow up on ideas or suggestions and resolve any questions or inconsistencies. The results should be compiled and reviewed by the decision group.

If time permits

Additional time can be spent on identifying system strengths, weaknesses, and desired improvements. If a significant project is being considered for replacing or upgrading an existing system, documentation for this project should begin here. A cost and benefit analysis for existing systems should also be conducted. Frequently, this analysis brings to light a great deal of information concerning the status of existing systems. It is common with these analyses that immediate operational improvements are required. If so, be sure to document any improvements to comply with the improving organizational performance section of the survey.

The above activity addresses the following IM standards:
- *IM.1 is addressed because this activity identifies the systems and requirements for internal and external data generation, and looks at the cost-effectiveness of various technologies.*

- *IM.6 may be addressed because this activity helps to document that the facility has internal and external database linkage.*

- *IM.9 will be addressed because this activity will show the need to link internal and external databases.*

4. Confirm the information budget and organization constraints

At a minimum
Gather the operating and capital budgets for information projects in all departments for the current year. Make sure you include staffing costs and an organization chart for information functions. Compile comparative numbers for the last several years and present this material to the decision group along with a range of changes for the next one to two years. Have the CFO review this material before the presentation. The goal of this activity is for the decision group to offer direction concerning financial constraints related to the hospital's business and financial situation. Do not include the costs or benefits of specific system projects in this presentation.

If time permits
Compare your hospital's information budget to other hospitals' budgets of similar size and service to determine if information projects are feasible. But, be careful not to skew this information for the presentation to the decision group. You will save time and effort by determining what information projects fit into the hospital's budget before an elaborate plan is developed, sent to the governing board, and declined. The point here is not to propose a project that costs more than the hospital can afford.

The above activity addresses IM.1 by showing that potential information projects are given direction as to their scope and complexity.

5. Establish ground rules for prioritizing projects

At a minimum
Establish ground rules for setting priorities. Explain these ground rules to the decision group and get its approval. To determine appropriate projects, use a rating system to weigh priorities, such as Nominal Group Technique or a decision matrix (see **Chapter 4**), and determine a set of attributes for each information need. The attributes should range from benefits, such as improved patient care and operating cost reductions, to added costs and any disruptions involved with implementing solutions. A priority scale should be used, such as an immediate need, an immediate need without time requirements, or a need that would be "nice to have."

If time permits
More elaborate ground rules can be designed if your hospital has time to do so. Additional attributes, analyses, and specifics concerning costs and benefits could also be researched. The primary objective of this activity is to create a means to measure needs and projects before expectations are raised, and to get a consensus on projects. By prioritizing the most important information projects and giving an explanation, the hospital will avoid the frustrated and angry feelings of those who wanted particular projects implemented.

Identify future needs and uses for information ——————————

When you have defined an information baseline, the next step is to get the organization to discuss its future needs and uses for information. Three major activities that will help do this are:

1. Consider opportunities for improvement for current systems,

2. Identify information needs that are not met by current systems, and

3. Develop information project descriptions that will help improve organizational performance.

1. Consider opportunities for improvement for current systems

At a minimum

Identify any major shortcomings of the hospital's current information systems. Recommend solutions for each problem and estimate the costs and difficulties involved. Even if it is not possible to fix the problem right away, be sure to state the costs involved as well as any benefits from improving it. Compile the information into a schedule for improvement and present it to the decision group. At this point, the decision group should understand the status of current systems so that efforts can be prioritized when it comes time for setting strategies.

If time permits

Consider user interviews on current systems as another resource for information. If the hospital has time, it could add details to documentation and include recommended solutions. Although visible or damaging problems may get immediate attention as a result of this activity, be careful not to get so focused on one project that you neglect other important new projects.

The above activity addresses the following standards:
- *IM.1 is addressed because this activity makes hospitals look for opportunities to improve performance.*
- *IM.8 is addressed because documentation generated in this activity can be used to show that performance improvement activities were conducted.*

2. Identify information needs that are not met by current systems

At a minimum

As part of researching opportunities for improvement for current systems, document users' requests for new or expanded system features that will require more information than is currently being collected. Review these results with the decision group. This activity can be combined with the previous one, but if a new system is being contemplated, this activity will be more compelling if done separately.

If time permits

Include a more thorough analysis of costs, benefits, and uses of new information. In the event a major new systems project or expenditure of funds is under consideration, make every effort to educate the decision group on the details of the project.

The above activity addresses IM.4 because it emphasizes the education of those who are making decisions regarding information systems in the hospital.

3. Develop information project descriptions

At a minimum
Group all the information gathered in the last two activities and create workable project descriptions. Each description should include a statement of benefits, costs, resources required, and scheduling considerations. These project descriptions will be a valuable resource when strategies and priorities are determined.

If time permits
Expand the project descriptions by including detailed information from system vendors, visits to other hospitals, or a more detailed cost and benefit analysis. Much of this analysis will be required before a major system project is implemented.

The above activity addresses IM.1 because it encourages the analysis of costs and benefits of technologies and systems. It also stresses the importance of communicating with customers, understanding their needs, and seeking out comparable information.

Develop information strategies ———————————————

The groups assigned to the information management project should have conducted detailed information-gathering and analysis. Before moving on to priority-setting and creating a schedule for implementation, consider the hospital's five information strategies, which are:
1. Patient records strategy,

2. Integration strategy,

3. Information systems and technology strategy,

4. Emergency preparedness strategy, and

5. Library services strategy.

For each of these information strategies, consider strategic information choices and identify any negative implications. Present this material to the decision group for approval. The results should be documented and kept for surveyors. The preparation of information management policies in the next section will be simplified by reviewing these strategies.

1. Patient records strategy

At a minimum

Define the scope and organization of patient records and include such factors as:
- cross-facility records access,
- ambulatory records management and access,
- referred diagnostic testing records,
- medication records management,
- guidelines for department-specific records, and
- the level of automation.

While some of these factors may be straightforward, others can have far-reaching implications and will need careful analysis and thoughtful consideration by the decision group.

If time permits

Add more detail to the definition of the patient records strategy, such as schematics for open and closed records, flow charts, and where major changes in approach are contemplated. Additional analysis could be done if the decision group decides on significant changes to the strategy.

The above activity addresses the following standards:
- *IM.1 is addressed because this activity allows for medical records assessment and direction and reviews its scope and complexity.*
- *IM.7 is addressed because this activity looks at the needs of the patient record.*

2. Integration strategy

At a minimum

Document the current level of system and information integration in the hospital and indicate any major planned changes. Integration refers to the gathering, sharing, and use of data across different systems to ensure consistency and accuracy. This activity will help if lack of integration causes problems or if integration will be addressed by a future project. One way to document current integration capabilities is to develop a Sources and Uses Table (see figure 3.2).

If time permits
Add more information to the analysis by considering integration-related barriers to improvement, priorities for change, and an overall approach to guiding future projects with regard to system and information integration. A more detailed analysis of current integration capabilities can be done by creating an Integration Capability Table (see figure 3.3).

The above activity addresses IM.6 and IM.9 because it addresses the need to integrate data as well as knowledge-based systems throughout the hospital.

3. Information systems and technology strategy

At a minimum
Document the hospital's approach to the five aspects of systems and technology and secure approval from the decision group. For each aspect, answer the questions, "How do we do this?" and "What standards do we adhere to?" The five aspects are:
- acquisition of application software;
- system software environment;
- hardware acquisition (regardless of size or location);
- voice and data communication; and
- organization for system development, installation, and operation.

If time permits
There is a vast amount of information and analysis that can be done to assess these five aspects of systems and technology. To narrow it down, focus on those areas that are controversial, problematic, or expecting major change as a result of the information project. Offer facts, options, and alternatives as needed.

The above activity addresses IM.1 and IM.3 because it analyzes the various types of technologies available to the hospital, as well as assesses its needs. IM.5 and IM.6 may also be addressed if the analysis includes a review of the different types of data generated by these systems with attention to timeliness and integration.

Figure 3.2

Sources and Uses Table

Information Sources	Administration/Registration	Physicians	Nurses	Ancillary services	Infection Control	Quality management	Safety and risk management	Senior administration/ Department directors	Finance	Medical staff services	Housekeeping	Dietary services	Referring physicians	Home care/ Aftercare agencies	Regulatory agencies
Medical record															
Patient demographics															
History & Physical															
Assessments															
- MD															
- RN															
- Social work															
- Etc.															
Diagnostic results															
- Lab															
- Pathology															
- Radiology															
Patient consent forms															
Advance directives															
Medication profile															
Op notes															
Discharge summary															
Information systems															
Patient demographics															
Insurance profile															
Diagnosis															
Procedures															
Detail charges															
Cost per case															
Library															
Clinical research papers															
Management literature															
Medline															
Other sources															
Department records															

Users

Use the chart to determine where information comes from and who uses it. Place a **S**, **U**, or **S/U** in the in the appropriate column.

S = Source of data   **U** = User of data   **S/U** = Both a source and user of data

Figure 3.3

Integration Capabilities Table

Information Types Search by:	Patient demographics	Date of service/LOS	Diagnosis	DRG	Procedures	Case type/acuity	Costs per case	Payer	Detail charges	Clinical service	Physician - Attending - Consulting - Referring - Group	Clinical outcome	Medication use	Equipment/Medical device	Incidents/Indicators

To get: Patient demographics, Date of service/LOS, Diagnosis, DRG, Procedures, Case type/acuity, Costs per case, Payer, Detail charges, Clinical service, Physician - Attending - Consulting - Referring - Group, Clinical outcome, Medication use, Equipment/Medical device, Incidents/Indicators

Determine the hospital's integration, search, and access capabilities by placing an **A**, **I**, or **M** in the appropriate box. For example, if you have a diagnosis for pneumonia and need to access the information on related procedures, record how that would be done on the chart.

A = Automated data access   **I** = Inquiry possible from same location   **M** = Manual compilation required

4. *Emergency preparedness strategy*

At a minimum
Define and document the hospital's approach to emergencies, such as those that result in the loss of voice or data communications, automated data systems, or critical hard copy records. Identify the plan for short- and long-term replacement of these systems and any records that are designated as critical. Your hospital-wide plan should include specific emergency procedures for each department.

If time permits
Expand this strategy to include other possible emergencies, more detailed priorities, and assignment of responsibilities.

The above activity addresses IM.2 because it assesses the need to prevent damage or loss to records.

5. *Library services strategy*

At a minimum
Define, document, and secure the approval of the decision group for at least the following:
- scope and focus of any in-house libraries,
- lending relationships,
- on-line services,
- subscription services,
- reference databases, and
- approaches to surveying users' needs.

If time permits
Consider using external bulletin boards, e-mail, and faxed services or subscriptions to enhance the hospital's information services.

The above activity addresses IM.9 because it analyzes the hospital's knowl-edge-based information resources.

Establish information management policies ——————————

The following policies are the core policies the hospital will need in order to address the IM standards. The working group will need to identify existing policies and may also have to draw up new policies and get them approved by the decision group. When all policies have been completed, collect them in a binder or folder to make index reference easier for surveyors.

The hospital should have a policy concerning each of the following areas or situations:
- mission statement for information management services;
- confidentiality and access to sensitive information within the organization and medical staff;
- release of medical records information, including
   ♦ who can request information internally and externally;
   ♦ what patient approval is needed;
   ♦ what information can be released, to whom, and in what form;
   ♦ who approves requests for information; and
   ♦ who is responsible for this policy and any exceptions;
- release of information to news media, including who is allowed to receive information and who authorizes the information;
- retention of medical records and other patient information;
- system development life cycle;
- purchase of computer hardware, software, and services;
- departmental and end-user computing;
- database administration; and
- information system availability, such as
   ♦ planned and unplanned downtime,
   ♦ hierarchy of applications, and
   ♦ continuous power commitments.

Completion of the above policies will address IM.1, IM.2, IM.3, IM.8, IM.9, and IM.10.

Set priorities and create an implementation plan ————————

With research and analysis completed and all necessary information policies written and approved, the final steps for the working and decision groups are to prioritize identified projects and to create a plan to begin implementation. There are three steps in this process:
   1. Estimate project time and the resources required,

2. Review the priorities of projects and select those to be implemented, and

3. Draft an implementation plan.

1. Estimate project time and the resources required

At a minimum

It is important for priority-setting and scheduling purposes to make at least an initial estimate of the time each project will require and the major resources involved. Consider staff time, cost of the project, and how existing systems will be affected. Use the experience of vendors or other organizations that have implemented similar projects as a basis for estimating time and resources. Allow a cushion in your schedule based on your organization's level of experience.

If time permits

Recruit selected staff members who work with the systems under consideration for improvement or who are affected by changes to be part of the project. This will give the working and decision groups feedback on what will or will not work. All staff involved in the information project should be given help with their other responsibilities.

The above activity addresses IM.1 because it identifies the need to plan for information management projects.

2. Review the priorities of projects and select those to be implemented

At a minimum

Using the rating system and the project descriptions set up earlier in this chapter, rate the projects selected for possible implementation. This iterative activity can be very political and interesting—especially when it comes to deciding on the winning projects (early implementation) and the losing ones (implementation in five years). Spend as much time as necessary to secure the understanding and approval of the decision group for granting top priorities to the next three or four projects to be implemented or those projects that will be addressed during the next 18 months.

If time permits

To be certain that the projects chosen will be most beneficial to the hospital, interview the users of those systems under consideration for improvement. Incorporate their comments and suggestions into the proposal and present it to the decision group.

3. Draft an implementation plan

At a minimum
With the assistance of the decision group and with the information gathered from research, draft a multiproject implementation plan. This plan should include project descriptions, project work plans, schedules, and the resources required to implement top priority projects. By grouping the projects into one plan, the decision group will be able to determine how projects overlap and to stagger their start and completion dates. Make sure to resolve any conflicts at this time so that the implementation of the project will be smooth. When the plan is completed, present it to the decision group for approval, who will, in turn, present it to the board and the medical staff.

If time permits
Use a project control system with a critical path analysis to add credibility to the plan. Project control systems generally include charts and graphs or an interactive display of task dependencies and target dates.

The above activity addresses IM.1 because it creates a plan for the implementation of information management projects.

Chapter 4

The Documentation Improvement Project

Chapter 4
The Documentation Improvement Project

Clinical information recorded in medical records is a key component of the JCAHO's accreditation process. Not only do the information management standards call for basic medical records documentation, but other standards do as well. The medical record is still the primary evidence a hospital has to show it follows its own policies, procedures, and mission.

This documentation improvement project focuses on the standards that rely on medical records content—and on the challenge of getting physicians to provide the documentation. It describes an ongoing review process for open and closed records. Forms and criteria for ongoing records review are included, as are practical ideas to help medical records managers facilitate better documentation. Finally, this project demonstrates how ongoing records review can fit into the hospital's overall strategies for performance improvement.

The benefits of a documentation improvement project are many. Improving documentation often means improving patient care through better communication—or at minimum, giving a clearer picture of the care a hospital is providing. For the purposes of JCAHO accreditation, a documentation improvement project gives the hospital a chance to compare its records and comply with standards for ongoing medical records review. Because this project is designed to follow performance improvement (PI) methods, hospitals can include it as one of its performance improvement activities.

The process for an ongoing records review program is the same as other PI activities and can be summarized by four general steps:
- ◆ Define the problem;
- ◆ Assess its causes and extent;
- ◆ Determine appropriate actions and implement them; and
- ◆ Monitor actions or solutions to ensure continuous quality.

The flow chart shown in figure 4.1 displays the process graphically.

Figure 4.1

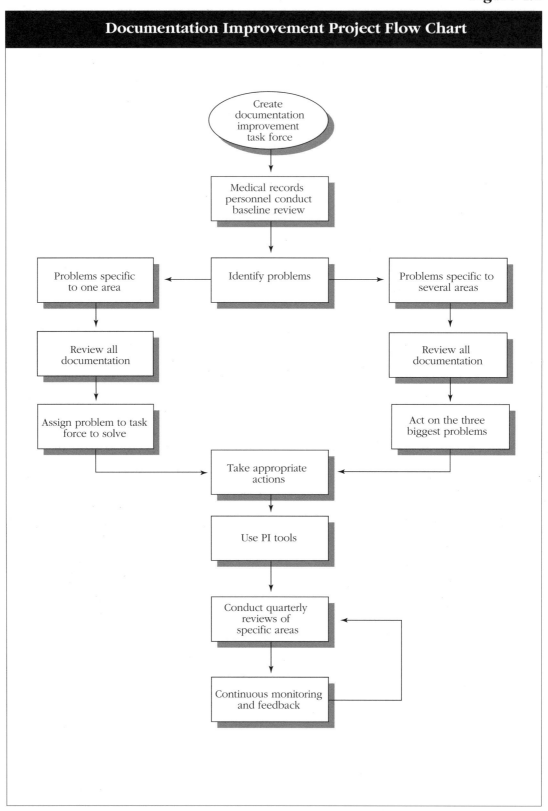

Documentation Improvement Project Flow Chart

Define the problem ——————————————————————————

One of the basic principles of PI is to make decisions based on data—not on instinct, perceptions, or suspicions. Therefore, to determine how well your hospital's medical records meet JCAHO standards, the first step is to obtain baseline data on current documentation practices.

The group primarily responsible for assessing documentation problems is usually the medical records committee, another existing committee, or a PI team created specifically for documentation improvement. In this chapter, the group will be called the documentation improvement task force, which should review problems with documentation, find the best ways to solve them, and then monitor their improvement.

The task force should include several members of the medical staff, the medical records director, a representative from nursing, and one additional person, if needed. The size of the group should be fewer than seven members to improve group dynamics and commitment. It is likely that the medical records director and his or her staff will provide the task force with professional input and technical support, including reviewing medical records for the baseline review and for subsequent reviews.

The baseline review

Before assessing problems, it's the job of the task force to determine where problems are by conducting a baseline review of a random sample of medical records. To obtain baseline data, compare an adequate random sample of records (see chart below) to all JCAHO documentation standards. To facilitate this review, use Figure 4.2 (located in **Appendix B**), which contains a listing of standards and provides 10 columns to document each record's compliance. It is important that enough records are included in this baseline review to make the results meaningful.

Number of discharges per year	Number of records in random sample
<2,000	50
2,000–5,000	100
>5,000	150

The sample should be random. One way to do so is to pick a time frame and a terminal digit and retrieve 50 to 150 completed records. This random sample of records does not have to include every physician or service. The ongoing review during the regular monitoring will take care of this important detail.

Such a project admittedly requires staff time and effort, yet it is an important component of preparing for the JCAHO's emphasis on medical records documentation. One comprehensive review will provide the information needed to perform smaller, less time-consuming reviews of problem areas throughout the year. But, if a department is unable to conduct a large-scale baseline review—and if a JCAHO survey is not imminent—it is possible to divide the review into monthly or quarterly increments.

Once the baseline review is completed, total the number of records meeting each standard and calculate a percentage of total records reviewed. Complete figure 4.3 (located in **Appendix B**). The first column of the worksheet shows the standard; the second and third show the percentage of records that must contain the documentation in order to score at least a 1 or 2. The documentation improvement task force should decide, in advance, whether it wants records compared to the criteria for a score of 1 or 2. In the fourth column, put the percentage of records meeting the standard and in the fifth column, place a 1, 2, N (for noncompliance), or NA (not applicable) to indicate the compliance of the record with the standard.

The medical records committee, department, or staff may want to provide historical data on previous records completion problems, including physicians, diagnoses, or procedures that most often cause records completion challenges. Such data will help the task force assess whether problems are recent or long term.

Assess the extent of documentation problems ————————————

The documentation improvement task force should review the completed baseline data display sheet (figure 4.3). Depending on the findings and the facility's own organizational setup, the task force may wish to take one or more of the following actions:

- ◆ For every standard in which documentation is inadequate, complete the sixth column in figure 4.3. Assign general responsibilities for documentation compliance to areas such as nursing and specific clinical or ancillary departments. Aggregate the documentation problems by group responsible and assign those groups the task of developing solutions and reporting back to the task force. See figure 4.4 for an example of a completed form.

♦ The task force may decide to review documentation problems differently by assigning responsibilities to other cross-functional teams for improvement activities. For example, a team responsible for the patient assessment standards may be given the responsibility of correcting documentation weaknesses related to patient assessment.

♦ If the documentation improvement task force finds serious documentation problems across the board, it may need to spend a month or more conducting a comprehensive review of the processes, forms, policies, procedures, incentives, and methods that lead to incomplete medical records.

♦ The documentation improvement task force should choose the most important or pervasive problems to work on. For example, the task force may find that three problems, such as lack of signatures, incomplete but timely discharge summaries, or lack of evidence that restraint policies are followed, cause 80% of the documentation deficiencies.

Determine appropriate actions and implement them ——————

Determining the underlying causes of documentation omissions is the next step in the documentation improvement process. Regardless of the organizational method the facility uses to assess documentation problems, it is important that each group look for the real causes of problems rather than assign blame or responsibility. Poorly designed forms, lack of time or physical space, misunderstood directions, and failure to understand the need for data may all cause incomplete documentation.

Quality improvement techniques are useful when assessing processes for improvement. The documentation improvement task force may want to use all or a combination of the following QI tools[†].

---

†See *Quality Improvement Techniques for Medical Records* for more information on quality improvement tools and techniques. **Appendix A** has more detail.

Figure 4.4

Medical Records Analysis Worksheet

JCAHO Standards	% required to score a 1	% required to score a 2	% of records with the documentation	Place a score of 1, 2, or N (non-compliance) or NA (not applicable)	Who is responsible for documenting the information?	Comments
PE.1.7—There is an H&P, indicated on diagnostic tests, and a pre-operative diagnosis on the record before surgery is performed (with the exception of emergencies).	100%	95–99%	80%	N	Surveyors	20% were late by one day
PE.1.7.1—There is a preanesthesia assessment for patients for whom anesthesia is planned.	100	95–99	96	2	Anesthesia staff	
PE.1.7.2—If anesthesia is planned, a licensed independent practitioner with appropriate clinical privileges determines if the patient is an appropriate candidate.	100	95–99	98	2	Anesthesia staff	
PE.1.7.3—If anesthesia is administered, the patient is re-evaluated immediately prior to anesthesia induction.	90–100	75–89	75	2	Anesthesia staff	
PE.1.7.4—The patient's status is assessed on admission to and discharge from the post-anesthesia recovery area.	90–100	75–89	69	N	Anesthesia staff	Dr. #1765 was responsible for 80% of the omissions

Brainstorming

Brainstorming is used to generate ideas on a specific subject or problem, for example, on the reasons for insufficient details in histories and physicals. It can be done in a group, using an unstructured discussion, or individually. All ideas are written down without thought to their logic or merit. A group can most effectively use brainstorming if the problem has to do with a system, process, or management use.

Nominal Group Technique (NGT)

Nominal Group Technique is similar to brainstorming but incorporates a rating system into the group discussion. All participants generate ideas and then rate them to determine the most important item to improve.

Customer satisfaction survey

A customer satisfaction survey is used to collect feedback on a system, process, or activity, such as the hours the medical records department is open and the services it offers physicians as they complete records. It is sent to the internal and external customers of a department, service, or area. The information in the survey generates important data that can be used with other QI tools, such as a cause and effect diagram, Pareto chart, or run chart.

Flow chart

A flow chart is used to identify all the steps in a process from start to finish, including all activities performed, decisions made, waiting periods, and documentation needed. A flow chart might be useful to follow the processes for dictating, transcribing, filing, and signing discharge summaries. It can be used as a pictorial representation of the activities or procedures within a department or area, such as the records analysis and completion process within the medical records department. A flow chart uses a standard set of symbols (circles, squares, diamonds, and arrows) that represent the various steps in a process.

Cause and effect diagram

A cause and effect diagram is used to identify the problems in a process, and is often used to structure the thoughts from a brainstorming session. It is commonly referred to as a fishbone diagram because of its shape, or the Ishikawa diagram after the person who refined the idea. It can be a simple or complex diagram.

Check sheet

A check sheet determines how often an event occurs. Data can be tallied to identify problems and their causes or to see patterns in a process that need to be changed. The check sheet is often a preliminary step for other QI tools, such as a Pareto chart, histogram, or run chart. Figure 4.2 used in the baseline review is an example of a check sheet.

Decision matrix

A decision matrix is a simple grid chart used to evaluate, compare, and seek out alternative solutions to a problem. The matrix works with preselected criteria (a standard against which to rate solutions or problems) and potential alternatives (solutions or problems). A group of people use the matrix to rate different alternatives to determine which one holds the highest priority. For example, a matrix may rate which of several changes to the records completion process would bring the most benefit to timely documentation and quality patient care.

Pareto chart

The Pareto chart is a bar graph that uses data to determine priorities in problem solving. It focuses on the priorities in a department or area, narrows down the causes of a problem, and illustrates how things may affect one another. Using horizontal and vertical axes, the causes of a problem and its frequency are plotted in the order of the largest to the smallest amounts of data.

Histogram

A histogram is a bar graph that displays data over time. It is used to search for problems or changes in a system or process. A histogram is based on raw data, such as numbers of delinquent records, that determine how the graph will be structured; unlike the Pareto chart, data remain in the order it is obtained. A check sheet should be used to gather the data.

Run chart

A run chart is a simple, plotted chart of data that shows the progress of a process over time. By analyzing the chart, trends, shifts, or changes in a process become evident. The chart tracks the time frame and the number of occurrences. Data is gathered from sources that are particular to a process and each set of data must be related in order for them to work together.

Scatter diagram

A scatter diagram shows possible relationships between two variables and how they interact with one another. It requires specific data collection to test the way one variable changes the other. The scatter diagram does not provide solutions—it only helps to test theories between variables. Other QI tools are needed to research the relationships in detail, such as brainstorming or a cause and effect diagram.

Searching for the cause of documentation problems is the same as searching for the solution. Armed with the knowledge of why the documentation isn't getting done, the team or committee assigned to the problem will have a much easier time identifying the appropriate actions to take. Figure 4.5 shows a number of conventional and unconventional ideas that hospitals have used to improve specific documentation problems.

Organizing and documenting is important to determine appropriate actions and implement them. This preparation forms the basis for the regular monitoring of solutions to ensure improvement. Regular monitoring allows the documentation improvement task force to pinpoint specific problems, make sure every physician is included in reviews, and focus its time and efforts.

Figure 4.6 helps the task force list documentation problems and assign responsibility for their study and solution. Complete the columns on the form as causes and solutions are identified. The last three columns are for monitoring the problem and will show which ones need to be followed-up in quarterly reviews.

Monitor to ensure continuous quality ————————————————

The last step in this documentation improvement project is regular monitoring. Ongoing reviews that are focused on problem areas found in the baseline review help to identify and document continuous problems. Structured appropriately, ongoing reviews will serve more than one need. The following discussion lists some of the added survey benefits that can be obtained from quarterly reviews.

Continuous quality improvement

To meet the primary and most important objective of this entire project—ongoing improvement of medical records documentation—it is important to make sure the project focuses on problem areas found in the baseline review.

Figure 4.5

Ideas to Improve Documentation †

Action	Examples	Problems it may correct	Pros	Cons
Develop and/or change policies and bylaws	◆ Implement more stringent medical staff bylaws governing records completion ◆ Develop policies covering patient care areas with documentation assignments ◆ Cooperate with neighboring hospitals to create consistent policies	Physicians or other staff members are not aware of their responsibilities or no one is assigned the responsibility.	By assigning responsibilities, it will be clear who is responsible for specific documentation activities.	Without staff reinforcement or taking care of other problems, such as form redesign, required documentation may continue to be overlooked.
Incentives	◆ Special events ◆ Providing food ◆ Drawings or contests ◆ Publicity for good documentation habits	Physicians and other staff members are aware of documentation requirements but lack sufficient motivation to carry them out.	Incentives often work, especially in motivating providers to complete backlogs. Cost may be minimal compared to improving reimbursement.	Some people see incentives as not addressing the real problem, essentially rewarding physicians and others for required activities.
Disincentives	◆ Suspension for delinquent records ◆ Restriction of admission or other privileges ◆ Fines ◆ Negative publicity ◆ Withholding other perks ◆ Calling physician to appear before the medical executive committee	Physicians and other staff members are aware of documentation requirements but lack sufficient motivation to carry them out.	These traditional methods may receive better acceptance by the medical staff than more innovative ones. If applied consistently, they will usually succeed. Using these methods requires good bookkeeping on the part of medical records staff; other direct costs are minimal.	Disincentives, especially restricting admitting or surgical privileges, could hurt the hospital financially more than help it with documentation compliance. Disincentive programs also require a substantial effort in monitoring completion, sending notices, restricting privileges, and communicating with physicians.

continued

† *For more information on records completion ideas, see Appendix A, pages 77–78*

Figure 4.5 cont.

Ideas to Improve Documentation

Action	Examples	Problems it may correct	Pros	Cons
Education/ reminders	◆ Inservices ◆ Reminders in medical records ◆ Pocket-sized reminders ◆ Posters at dictation areas or in other parts of the hospital	Physicians and other staff are not aware of documentation requirements, forget them, or fail to understand their importance.	Educational efforts are usually well accepted, non-offensive, and complement physicians' desire to do their jobs well. Education may also help with the detail and timeliness of documentation.	Without reinforcement or continuous reminders, physicians may forget certain requirements. Education by itself may not motivate physicians to improve documentation.
Forms	◆ Better designed forms to facilitate documentation completion ◆ Checklists as part of form function as a reminder	Physicians and other staff are not aware of or forget about documentation requirements.	Well designed forms encourage accurate documentation.	Well designed forms may not help with the timeliness of documentation. Redesigning forms may be a large-scale and time-consuming effort.
Computers	◆ Electronic signatures ◆ Online records completion ◆ Point-of-care data capture ◆ Faxing copies of signed reports	Documentation requirements take too much time or are burdensome.	Depending on the programs and the willingness of users to learn them, computers can make documentation easier.	Computers, software, and other additions can be expensive projects. Equipment goals can often become more important than improvements in documentation.
Other equipment improvements	◆ Improve dictation system or retrain medical staff ◆ Provide loaner or portable dictation units for physicians to use outside the hospital	Documentation requirements take too much time or are burdensome.	Depending on the programs and the willingness of users to learn them, certain equipment can make documentation easier.	Equipment improvements does not remedy lack of knowledge of what to document or motivation to provide details.

continued

Figure 4.5 cont.

Ideas to Improve Documentation

Action	Examples	Problems it may correct	Pros	Cons
Environmental or physical space changes	◆ Redesign nursing unit to ensure quiet place for records completion ◆ Leave record on unit for a specified period of time for completion ◆ Make medical record department's record completion area more comfortable ◆ Create delivery service to take records to physicians or place them in a central area in the hospital for completion	Environmental barriers impede records completion, even if there is motivation to do so.	If motivation to document is present, changes in the physical layout of records completion areas may be beneficial.	Environmental improvements does not provide knowledge of what to document or motivation to provide details.
Change attitudes toward record completion	◆ Monitor trends in documentation rather than for individual deficiencies ◆ Encourage an attitude that supports documentation as part of patient care ◆ Create a review program that checks documentation on nursing units concurrently with care being given	Physicians do not complete records without pressure, monitoring, and follow up from the hospital.	Changes in attitudes puts the responsibility for documentation on those who are supposed to provide it. It may also reduce work and change the image of the medical records department.	Hospitals may determine that attitude improvement programs do not provide adequate control to ensure that hospital goals for documentation are met. Legal questions may arise if physicians fail to take the challenge and provide complete documentation.

Figure 4.6

Medical Records Review Tracking Form						
Documentation problem and related standards	Group responsible for analysis	Causes	Actions to correct problem	When to re-review?	Results of re-review	Ongoing monitoring plan

If the baseline review revealed numerous problems across several areas, it may be easier to set a longer timetable of reviews (see figure 4.7).

Figure 4.7

Agenda of Ongoing Reviews

September 1997	◆ Baseline review
October 1997	◆ Actions taken to improve documentation
November 1997	◆ Re-review 20 records of Dr. # 1765 to determine if PE.1.7.4 is met ◆ Review 50 records of patients currently hospitalized for PE.1.6.1 to determine if new transcription service has 24-hour turnaround ◆ Review 20 records of patients receiving parenteral nutrition to ensure that TX.4 is met
December 1997	◆ Re-review 20 surgery records of Dr. # 1765 to determine if PE.1.7.4 is met ◆ Review 50 surgery records to determine if TX.2.1 is met ◆ Review 50 records at random to ensure IM.3.2.1.1 is documented
January 1998	◆ Re-review 20 surgery records of Dr. #1765 to determine if PE.1.7.4 is met ◆ Review 20 records at one week postdischarge to ensure that IM.7 is met
February 1998	◆ Re-review 20 surgery records of Dr. # 1765 to determine if PE.1.7.4 is met ◆ Review 20 podiatry records to ensure that MS.6.2.2 is met ◆ Review 50 records at random to ensure IM.3.2.1.1 is documented
March 1998	◆ Review 50 surgery records to determine if TX.2.1 is met ◆ Review 50 records at random to ensure IM.3.2.1.1 is documented
April 1998	◆ Review 20 podiatry records to ensure that MS.6.2.2 is met ◆ Review 50 records to ensure that PE.4.3, RI.1.2, and TX.1.2 are met

If documentation problems, found in the baseline review, were limited to certain areas, ongoing monitoring of those areas may be sufficient. Other, more focused reviews can be incorporated as problems arise, as JCAHO standards change, or when hospital documentation needs become more refined.

Ongoing medical records review

The ongoing medical records review can also show compliance with JCAHO standard IM.3.2.1 (often referred to as clinical pertinence review) if it meets the following JCAHO requirements:

- ◆ the review is conducted for completeness, accuracy, and timely completion of records;

- ◆ while records are reviewed by medical records or other staff assigned the job, analysis of the review is performed by the documentation improvement task force, medical records committee, or any other group of medical staff, nursing, medical record staff, management and administrative services, and representatives of other departments as needed;

- ◆ the review determines that a representative sample of records, defined as the organization's full scope of practice, includes the most common diagnoses, procedures, and high-risk procedures. At least one medical record from each physician on the medical staff should be included annually;

- ◆ the review addresses the presence, accuracy, timeliness, and authentication of the following items found in the medical record:
    - identification data;
    - medical history, including chief complaint, details of present illness, inventory by body systems, and relevant past, social, and family histories;
    - summary of the patient's psychosocial needs as appropriate;
    - report of relevant physical exam;
    - statement on conclusions from the history and physical;
    - statement on action planned for patient;
    - diagnostic and therapeutic orders;
    - evidence of appropriate informed consent;
    - clinical observations, including results of therapy;
    - progress notes made by the medical staff and other authorized staff;

- consultation reports;
- reports of operative and other invasive procedures, tests, and their results;
- reports of any diagnostic and therapeutic procedures, such as pathology and clinical laboratory examinations, radiology, and nuclear medicine;
- records of donations and receipt of transplants and implants;
- final diagnosis or diagnoses;
- conclusions at termination of hospitalization;
- discharge summaries;
- discharge instruction; and
- results of autopsy if performed;

- ◆ all the above aspects of the review must be documented in minutes or reports.

The JCAHO's performance improvement requirements

In its performance improvement (PI) standards, the JCAHO brings nearly every aspect of hospital care and every department into the performance improvement loop. The following standards emphasize that the ongoing monitoring and improvement of medical records documentation are vital components of a hospital's overall performance improvement program:

- ◆ PI.3—The hospital must have a process to collect data to measure important existing processes.

- ◆ PI.3.1—The hospital must measure the performance of patient care and organizational functions. Among the functions specifically mentioned in this standard are:
  - the appropriateness of surgery, preparing the patient and performing the procedures, and providing postprocedure care;
  - the use of medications, including prescribing and monitoring their effects;
  - the use of blood and its components, including ordering and monitoring its effects; and
  - information on autopsy results, dietetic, laboratory, radiology, nuclear medicine, radiation oncology services, and drug reactions.

- ◆ PI.4—The hospital must assess the collected data to determine whether existing processes are performed well, if processes need to be improved and how they can be improved, and if changes resulted in improvement.

The challenge here is to meet all these goals in an organized medical record review program. The baseline review and its identification of problems and actions is a key first step. Documenting the findings and identifying group responsibilities for reporting on actions taken is also important. The documentation improvement task force should schedule reviews for the next year (or the next two years if documentation problems are extreme and solutions are sophisticated) to make sure the effort is continuous and organized.

Conducting the ongoing review

For each review, the task force should identify a limited number of review criteria using, for example, the standards that were not being met in one particular area or one or two important pieces of documentation. Reviewers should use figure 4.8 to create a review form for the review focus.

Select an adequate sample of records for the review. The guidelines below suggest the number of records to include. It is also important for the review to include all physicians, common diagnoses, procedures, and high-risk procedures to meet IM.3.2.1. Figure 4.8 has a column to identify physicians or record their initials. The documentation improvement task force should make sure that at least one record for each physician is included throughout the course of a year, even if it means structuring the last review to cover a general category, such as late histories and physicals, in order to

Number of discharges per year	Number of records in review
<2,000	25*
2,000-5,000	50*
>5,000	75*

* In addition, include five open records selected and reviewed by utilization review, quality assurance, or medical records staff on patient units.

Figure 4.8

Ongoing Medical Records Review Worksheet

Topic: _____
Records to be included: _____
Reason records were chosen: _____

Documentation problem and related standard	% required for hospital compliance satisfaction	Did records meet standards?	Physician identification	Comments

include the records of the physicians who have not yet been reviewed.

Any time a review focuses on a general problem that crosses all diagnoses and procedures, such as late histories and physicals, choose records from a list of frequent diagnoses, procedures, or high-risk procedures. Be sure to document the reason for selecting these records at the top of the review form. It may also be useful for the task force to include a review of the items listed in IM.7 to ensure compliance with JCAHO standards.

The review's function is to present findings to the documentation improvement task force or its designee. To comply with IM.3.2.1, physicians and other personnel must participate in the review, but do not necessarily have to review every record that fails to meet a documentation criterion. Thus, the task force should set thresholds for when it should review records. For example, the task force might review a specific percentage of records each month or review the five worst records identified.

Analyzing the findings is the next step. Take action on the results and assign follow-up responsibilities with a time frame attached. As with the baseline review, it's important to identify the causes of the problem before determining the remedy.

In summary, preparing for the JCAHO's emphasis on the content of medical records is a critical part of survey preparation. Analyzing the status of medical records for compliance with JCAHO standards should be viewed as a positive quality improvement project. It is useful for improving documentation, demonstrating performance improvement, and meeting JCAHO requirements for medical records review.

Chapter 5

Preparing for Survey

Chapter 5
Preparing for Survey

Being prepared for the JCAHO survey process is more than just important—it's critical to your hospital's accreditation success. And in preparing for this survey, a change of direction is needed—away from a focus solely on documentation and toward preparing staff for interviews and the hospital for surveyor observations.

There are two aspects to succeeding with the survey process—getting into compliance and then demonstrating it. Compliance can only happen over time and with a multidisciplinary approach to meeting the intent of each standard. Then at survey time, the hospital can effectively demonstrate what's been done and what types of projects are in progress.

The survey process includes interviews and discussions with hospital leaders and staff. This chapter will help you prepare for the three major sessions that focus on IM as well as offer helpful advice on how to prepare other hospital staff who may not have a direct relationship to the IM standards but who must be prepared for surveyor questions. The three sessions are

- ◆ the document review session,
- ◆ the information management interview, and
- ◆ the medical record interview.

Take note that medical records will be reviewed during patient unit visits, also called open record review. IM standards are not particularly targeted during these sessions. However, hospital staff should be prepared to answer questions that may be related to information management during patient unit visits.

The document review session

Well in advance of its survey, a hospital will receive from the JCAHO a pre-survey package that explains what to expect at every point of the survey. This material includes a detailed list of documents to be provided for the two-hour document review session that begins the survey. The IM-specific documents that must be available for review are listed in figure 5.1.

What to expect

Surveyors use the document review session to identify various information they will use throughout the survey. Thus, hospitals should be meticulous in preparing their documents. All documents should be dated, timely, and current. The survey coordinator (the person assigned to organizing survey activities) should review IM-related documents to make sure they are up to date.

Surveyors will also look for proof that the hospital is doing what it has written down. The document review session provides the survey team with a strong impression of the hospital and helps them to later validate that impression through interaction and observation. The emphasis on documentation is especially important for the IM portion of the survey because of the JCAHO's focus on the medical record.

The IM standards and survey process emphasize the need to involve the right people in the right activities. Any collaboration among staff in information management–related activities should be highlighted in the documents provided for the surveyors.

What to do

To make it easier for the surveyors to review IM-related documentation, do the following:

- Assemble, organize, and label all IM-related documents.

- Make sure IM documents are properly cross-referenced in the main index for this session as outlined in the JCAHO presurvey package. Note where additional, supportive documentation can be found.

- Emphasize documentation that contains organization-wide policies for information management. All departments that are involved with information management should collaborate on policies.

- Document information management issues raised in meetings, actions taken, and results achieved to show that they were completed.

- Review IM-related documents before the survey to highlight communication and collaboration, especially if there was multidisciplinary involvement on information management projects.

Figure 5.1

List of Documents for the Document Review Session

IM.7

◆ All related policies on medical record content.

◆ Policies and procedures on advance directives.

◆ Policies and procedures on treatments or procedures that need informed consent documentation.

◆ Discharge information on medications prescribed and dispensed.

◆ Rules and regulations pertaining to medical staff verbal orders for medication and who authenticates them.

◆ Rules and regulations pertaining to verbal orders that pose potential hazards to patients.

◆ Policies and procedures related to the content and timely completion of medical records.

◆ Policies and procedures on entries in the medical record by house staff and who countersigns them.

◆ Policies and procedures related to the recording of operative reports.

◆ Policies and procedures related to patients who receive ambulatory care regularly.

◆ Policies and procedures related to patients who receive emergency treatment.

◆ Select a person or persons familiar with information management in the hospital to do a mock review of all IM-related documents. Have this person look to see that the cross-references in the index are accurate and that all IM documents are presentable and clearly labeled.

The information management interview ————————————————

The information management interview is conducted on the second day of the survey and focuses on assessing the hospital's information management planning and processes. The people who should attend are the CIO, information management director, resource center manager or librarian, medical records director, and other key people involved in information management, if needed.

What to expect
Surveyors will review the following topics:
- types of aggregate data used in the hospital;
- how aggregate data is used to support decisions and performance improvement activities;
- how information is made available to staff;
- how data is integrated within the hospital;
- how comparative data is used;
- how the confidentiality, security, and integrity of the patient record is maintained;
- who is responsible for information availability; and
- the kinds of data definitions and data capture methods used in the hospital.

Surveyors may discuss the following topics:
- policies on timely completion of records,
- availability of records,
- clinical pertinence of the record,
- the coding and retrieval system,
- information integration within the hospital,
- types of aggregate data used to support decisions,
- history and physical completion after admission,
- history and assessment of the patient if readmitted,
- timely autopsy results,
- use of comparative data, and
- the results of the hospital's closed medical record review.

What to do

To prepare for the information management interview, gather all the people who will take part and hold rehearsal sessions. Develop a list of mock questions based on the topics above and distribute them to attendees. Ask a person who is familiar with information management to act as surveyor/ moderator of the session.

After the session, the person who acts as moderator should critique individuals' answers and offer suggestions on the best way to answer a question—answers that are to the point and do not offer more information than is necessary.

Finally, even though surveyors will not focus on documentation during this session, it is a good idea to have key high-level documents available to support attendees' answers.

The medical record interview ————————————————————

The medical record interview is a survey activity that helps to assess the hospital's performance in documenting patient care. The records to be reviewed will be specified by the survey team on the first day of survey, after the document review session. Medical records staff then have to gather the required records (about 20), review them against a medical record review form, and tally the results. (See **Appendix C** for a checklist that reflects the JCAHO's review form.) The review will take place during the medical record interview by those in attendance. During the medical record review, each interview participant will match the information in the record against the requirements on the review form. The records requested may include psychiatry, obstetrics, surgery, emergency services, pediatrics, physical rehabilitation, and dental services.

The medical record interview will require that the following people attend: members from administration/management, the medical records director, medical records staff who reviewed the records, medical staff members, and nursing representatives. Representatives from groups such as the medical records committee should also attend this interview. It is extremely important that all those who attend are knowledgeable of the standards, the medical record, and the review form.

The JCAHO views the medical record review as a learning experience. Hospital staff who contribute to the patient record should be familiar with the content of the record, the hospital's format, and where to find information in the medical record. The review is intended to help the hospital identify problems in documenting care and opportunities for improvement.

It is important to obtain the most current version of the medical record review form before the survey, either from the JCAHO or from a recently surveyed hospital.

What to expect

The staff participating in the review will need to be familiar with and locate in the patient record the following IM-related items:
- legal representatives;
- verbal orders;
- dated entries;
- physician authentication;
- medical history and physical;
- diagnosis or impression;
- reasons for admission;
- treatment goals and plan;
- evidence of advance directives;
- evidence of informed consent;
- diagnostic and therapeutic orders and results;
- operative and other procedure notations;
- progress notes;
- documented clinical observations;
- documented response to care;
- consultation reports;
- prescribed or ordered medications;
- administered medications;
- prescribed medication upon discharge;
- documentation of donated and received transplants;
- autopsy results;
- all relevant diagnoses;
- external or internal care or community agency referral notations;
- discharge summary;
- unusual events or complications;
- operative reports written or dictated after surgery, authenticated, and operative progress noted immediately after surgery;

    - list of diagnoses, medications, conditions, allergies, and procedures for regularly seen ambulatory patients; and

    - policies and procedures related to emergency care patients.

What to do

To prepare for the medical record interview and review of records, complete the documentation improvement project in **Chapter 4** and train the people who will participate. Participants should be chosen carefully. The documentation improvement project will identify weaknesses in hospital documentation. This project instructs the hospital to improve the problems in documentation as best it can. Participants should be educated on any documentation problems and how they are being improved.

Educate participants on how to review the medical record in one or more rehearsal sessions. These sessions should cover how to locate all items in the medical record listed on the review form. To do this, gather participants together and distribute a sampling of records and a copy of the review form. Have all participants review the IM-related standards (as well as the others) on the review form with the record and encourage them to ask questions. Review the results of this mock review session to see if records are generally ready for JCAHO scrutiny.

On the day of the review, make sure all participants are supplied with a copy of the review form. To prepare the hospital to respond to possible Type I recommendations, consider pre-labeling the records selected for the session.

Interviews with hospital staff on IM standards ────────────

Surveyors will not limit the discussion of IM standards to just the IM interview or the medical record interview. Essentially, any hospital staff member is a potential candidate to answer questions on information management processes. In fact, since all areas of the hospital deal with information, nearly all staff members could have some sort of information management questions asked of them. Therefore, it is not only important to prepare information management staff and those attending specific IM-related meetings, it is equally important to extend that preparation and training to all staff.

Other individuals who will need training in information management are:
- CEO,
- CFO,
- other leaders of the hospital,
- all department directors,
- the quality improvement council (or equivalent),
- resource center services,
- nursing,
- pharmaceutical services,
- emergency and ambulatory care services,
- clinical laboratory services,
- dietetic services,
- imaging services,
- medical staff department and leadership,
- physical rehabilitation services,
- respiratory care services,
- social work services,
- special care units, and
- environment of care services.

What to expect

Surveyors will focus on various IM standards in different areas of the hospital. To be completely prepared, staff should be familiar with the IM standards related to their department's activities as well as the hospital's overall IM functions.

Surveyors will use a verbal approach when interviewing or gaining information on IM services from any area not specifically related to the creation or implementation of information. For example, the following list reviews a sampling of what areas or topics may be covered in a department or service. Use the list as a base for training, but remember, surveyors may ask questions related to other IM functions in addition to the ones mentioned here.

Leadership and CEO
 ◆ How IM services meet the needs of the organization
 ◆ The types of aggregate data used in decision-making

All department directors
 ◆ IM training and education

◆ Use of aggregate data in decision-making
◆ Use and availability of knowledge-based information

Medical staff and nursing
  ◆ Accessibility of the medical record
  ◆ Timeliness of diagnostic tests
  ◆ Types of aggregate data used in decision-making
  ◆ Access to knowledge-based information
  ◆ Format of the medical record
  ◆ Use of comparative data

Environment of care services
  ◆ Use of aggregate data

Pharmaceutical services
  ◆ Physician authentication
  ◆ Use of aggregate data
  ◆ DEA and poison control information
  ◆ Availability of hospital formulary

Resource center
  ◆ Accessibility and timeliness of knowledge-based information
  ◆ Use of external and internal databases
  ◆ Use of aggregate data

QI council (or equivalent)
  ◆ How IM processes are linked with patient care and hospital functions
  ◆ How data is used for performance improvement

Emergency and ambulatory care services
  ◆ The control register process

What to do
Plan a training session that includes the above mentioned individuals, groups, or departments. These sessions should include specifics on the information management processes in the departments and the hospital. Also consider using role-playing during the session.

Write and distribute a memo explaining when training sessions will be offered. Encourage all to attend and emphasize what the new survey changes mean to the hospital and why staff need to be prepared. If training sessions are not possible, prepare at least an outline of important information on IM services.

Appendix A
Resource Guide

Appendix A
Resource Guide

Organizations

American College of Healthcare Executives
1 North Franklin Street, Suite 1700
Chicago, IL 60606
Telephone: 312/424-2800
Fax: 312/424-0023
E-mail: *GenInfo@ache.org*
Website: *www.ache.org*
• Publishers of the *Healthcare Executive*

American Health Information Management Association (AHIMA)
919 North Michigan Avenue, Suite 1400
Chicago, IL 60611
Telephone: 312/787-2672
Fax: 312/787-9793
E-mail: *info@ahima.org*
Website: *www.ahima.org*
• Publishers of the *Journal of the American Health Information Management Association*
• Offers seminars on information management

Center for Healthcare Information Management (CHIM)
3800 Packard Road, Suite 150
Ann Arbor, MI 48108
Telephone: 313/973-6116
Fax: 313/973-6996
E-mail: *jpatters@chim.org*
Website: *www.chim.org*

College of Healthcare Information Management Executives (CHIME)
3300 Washtenaw Avenue
Ann Arbor, MI 48104
Telephone: 313/665-0000
Fax: 313/665-4922
E-mail: *info@chime-office.org*
Website: *www.chime-net.org*

Healthcare Information and Management Systems Society (HIMSS)
230 East Ohio Street, Suite 600
Chicago, IL 60611-3201
Telephone: 312/664-4467
Fax: 312/664-6143
E-mail: *himss@himss.org*
Website: *www.himss.org*
• Publishers of *Healthcare Information Management*

The Accreditation Resource
A division of The Greeley Company
100 Hoods Lane
Marblehead, MA 01945
Telephone: 781/639-8030
Fax: 781/639-2982
E-mail: *webmaster@opuscomm.com*
Website: *www.greeleycom/education/tar/tar.html*
• Consulting organization that offers seminars on JCAHO accreditation and information management

Books

Ball, Marion *et al.*, eds. *Health Information Management Systems: A Practical Guide.* New York: Springer-Verlag, 1991.

DeLuca, Joseph M. with Owen Doyle. *Health Care Information Systems: An Executive's Guide for Successful Management.* Chicago: American Hospital Publishing, 1991.

Healthcare Information and Management Systems Society. *Guide to Effective Health Care Information and Management Systems.* Chicago: HIMSS, 1994.

Mangano, Joseph J., ed. *Health Information Management—A Comprehensive Guide to Current Regulations and Management Practices.* Los Angeles: Practice Management Information Corporation, 1993.

Priest, Stephen L. *Understanding Computer Resources: A Healthcare Perspective.* Owing Mills: National Health Publishing, 1989.

Umbaugh, Robert E., ed. *Handbook of IS Management*, 3rd edition. Boston: Auerbach Publishers, 1991.

Handbook of IS Management, 1992-93 yearbook. Boston: Auerbach Publishers, 1992.

Periodicals ————————————————————————————

American Journal of Health-System Pharmacy
American Society of Health-System Pharmacists
7272 Wisconsin Avenue
Bethesda, MD 20849
Telephone: 301/657-3000
Fax: 301/657-1251
E-mail: *info@ashp.org*
Website: *www.ashp.org*

American Medical News
American Medical Association
515 North State Street
Chicago, IL 60610
Telephone: 312/464-5000
Fax: 312/464-4184
E-mail: *insight@ama-assn.org*
Website: *www.ama-assn.org*

Healthcare Financial Management
Healthcare Financial Management Association
2 Westbrook Corporate Center, Suite 700
Westchester, IL 60154
Telephone: 708/531-9600
Fax: 708/531-0032
Website: *www.hfma.org*

Healthcare Informatics
McGraw-Hill Company
1221 Avenue of the Americas
New York, NY 10020-1095
Telephone: 212/512-2000
E-mail: *aharste@mcgraw-hill.com*
Website: *www.healthcare-informatics.com*

Health Management Technology
Intertech Publishing
9800 Metcalf
Overland Park, KS 66212
Telephone: 913/341-1300
Fax: 913/967-1898
Website: *www.intertech.com*

Hospitals and Health Networks
American Hospital Publishing, Inc.
737 N. Michigan Avenue, Suite 700
Chicago, IL 60611
Telephone: 312/440-6800
Fax: 312/951-8491
E-mail: *webmaster@ahpi.inlet.com*
Website: *www.amhpi.com*

Information Week: The Newsmagazine for Information Management
CMP Publications, Inc.
600 Community Drive
Manhasset, NY 11030
Telephone: 516/562-5000
Website: *www.techweb.cmp.com/corporate/current/default.html*

Inside Healthcare Computing
Inside Information Group
3600 South Harbor Blvd., Suite 220
Oxnard, CA 93035
Telephone: 805/984-8500
Fax: 805/984-8504
Website: *insidehealth.com*

M.D. Computing
Springer-Verlag New York, Inc.
175 Fifth Avenue
New York, NY 10010
Telephone: 800/777-4643
Fax: 212/473-6272
Website: *www.springer-ny.com*

Modern Healthcare
Crain Communications, Inc.
740 N. Rush Street
Chicago, IL 60611-2590
Telephone: 312/649-5200
Fax: 312/280-3183
E-mail: *CLauer@crain.com*
Website: *crain.co.uk/crain-inc.html*

Opus Communications
P.O. Box 1168
Marblehead, MA 01945
Telephone: 781/639-1872
Fax: 781/639-2982
E-mail: *customer_service@opuscomm.com*
Website: *www.opuscomm.com*
Clinical Pertinence Review: Winning Strategies for Your JCAHO Survey
Mastering Medical Records Completion: Successful Strategies from Medical
  Records Briefing
Medical Records Briefing
Quality Improvement Techniques for Medical Records

The Quality Letter for Healthcare Leaders
Capitol Publications, Inc.
1101 King Street, Ste. 444
Alexandria, VA 22314
Telephone: 703/683-4100
Fax: 703/739-6517
E-mail: *webmaster@cappubs.com*
Website: *www.cappubs.com*

Quality Progress
American Society for Quality
611 East Wisconsin Avenue
Milwaukee, WI 53202
Telephone: 414/272-8575
Fax: 414/272-1734
Website: *www.asq.org*

The Joint Commission Journal on Quality Improvement
Joint Commission on Accreditation of Healthcare Organizations
One Renaissance Blvd.
Oakbrook Terrace, IL 60181
Telephone: 630/916-5800
Fax: 630/916-5644
E-mail: *cmyers@jcaho.org*
Website: *www.jcaho.org*

QRC Advisor
Topics in Health Information Management
Topics in Health Record Management
Aspen Publishers, Inc.
200 Orchard Ridge Drive
Gaithersburg, MD 20878
Telephone: 800/638-8437
Fax: 301/417-7650
Website: *www.aspenpub.com*

Appendix B
Chapter 4 Forms

Figure 4.2

Medical Records Review Worksheet

Note patient record numbers.

JCAHO Standard	Record:	1	2	3	4	5	6	7	8	9	10
Patient Rights (RI)											
RI.1, RI.1.2.3, RI.1.3.4—There is evidence of a resolved ethical or treatment issue.											
RI.1.1—The patient is admitted and/or transferred based on his or her need for services.											
RI.1.2—The patient and, when appropriate, the family is involved in the patient's care.											
RI.1.2.1–RI.3—Informed consent is obtained for treatments, or procedures, or research participants (benefits, risks, and alternatives are discussed).											
RI.1.2.2—If appropriate, surrogate decision-makers are identified.											
RI.1.2.4—The patient is asked if he or she has an advance directive, and if so, the advance directive is in the record, or the intent of the advance directive is documented.											
RI.1.2.5–RI.1.2.6—DNR and withholding or withdrawing life-sustaining treatment orders follow hospital policy.											

✓ -met   ✗ -failed   ( )-comments

Figure 4.2 cont.

Medical Records Review Worksheet

Note patient record numbers.

JCAHO Standard	Record: 1	2	3	4	5	6	7	8	9	10
RI.1.2.7—The patient and family members' needs are individually addressed during the end of life.										
RI.1.3.4—Patient and/or family complaints are addressed.										
RI.1.3.5—Requested pastoral counseling is provided.										
RI.1.3.6—Individual (non-English-speaking, visually or hearing impaired) patient communication needs are considered.										
RI.2—The procurement and donation of organs and other tissues follow organizational policy.										
Assessment of Patients (PE)										
PE.1—There is a physical, psychological, and social status assessment.										
PE.1.1—The scope and intensity of further assessments are based on diagnosis, the care setting, desire for care, and response to any previous treatment.										
PE.1.2—Nutritional status is assessed when indicated by the patient's needs.										
PE.1.3–PE.1.3.1—Functional status is assessed when indicated by the patient's needs (a must for patients referred for rehab services).										

✓-met   ✗-failed   ( )-comments

Figure 4.2 cont.

Medical Records Review Worksheet

Note patient record numbers.

JCAHO Standard	Record:	1	2	3	4	5	6	7	8	9	10
PE.1.4—Appropriate diagnostic tests are performed to determine any patient needs.											
PE.1.4.1—Records show requests for diagnostic tests provide adequate clinical information.											
PE.1.5—The need for a discharge planning assessment is determined.											
PE.1.6—The initial assessment is completed within the time set by hospital policy.											
PE.1.6.1—The H&P, nursing assessment, and other assessments are completed and recorded within 24 hours of admission for inpatients.											
PE.1.7—There is an H&P, indicated diagnostic tests, and a pre-operative diagnosis on the record before surgery is performed (with the exception of emergencies).											
PE.1.7.1—Preanesthesia assessment for patients for whom anesthesia is planned.											
PE.1.7.2—If anesthesia is planned, a licensed independent practitioner with appropriate clinical privileges determines if the patient is an appropriate candidate.											
PE.1.7.3—If anesthesia is administered, the patient is reevaluated immediately prior to anesthesia induction.											

✓ -met   ✗ -failed   ( )-comments

Figure 4.2 cont.

Medical Records Review Worksheet

Note patient record numbers.

JCAHO Standard	Record:	1	2	3	4	5	6	7	8	9	10
PE.1.7.4—The patient's status is assessed on admission to and discharge from the post-anesthesia recovery area.											
PE.1.9.1—Laboratory and pathology services and results are provided on a timely basis through the hospital's laboratories or an approved reference laboratory.											
PE.1.14.2—If patient is getting blood glucose monitored on unit, the results are traceable to the machine used for testing.											
PE.2—The patient is reassessed according to hospital policy.											
PE.2.2—Reassessment occurs at regular intervals and determines the patient's response to care.											
PE.2.3–PE.2.4—Patient is reassessed when there is a significant change in the patient's condition or diagnosis.											
PE.3—Patient needs are identified and prioritized.											
PE.3.1—Care decisions are based on identified patient needs and priorities.											
PE.4.2—For patients that need emergency care, assessments and treatment are determined by a LIP.											
PE.4.3—In areas where nursing care is provided, an RN assesses the patient's nursing care needs.											

✓ -met ✗ -failed ( )-comments

Figure 4.2 cont.

Medical Records Review Worksheet

Note patient record numbers.

Record:	1	2	3	4	5	6	7	8	9	10
JCAHO Standard										
PE.5—Infants, children, or adolescent patients are individually assessed for psychosocial needs, development aspects, immunizations, family, or guardian expectations and involvement for treatment.										
PE.6—Emotionally or behaviorally disordered patients are individually assessed for their history of mental, emotional, behavioral, and substance abuse problems, a mental status examination, problem behaviors, and a psychosocial assessment.										
PE.7—Substance abuse patients are individually assessed for history of alcohol or drug use, physical problems associated with abuse, family history of substance abuse, spiritual orientation, previous treatment, response to previous treatment, history of physical or sexual abuse, sexual history and orientation.										
PE.8—Patients of suspected abuse or neglect are identified, appropriate consents are obtained, and legally required notifications occurred.										
Treatment of Patients (TX)										
TX.1—Records show that the care, treatment, and rehabilitation plans are appropriate and individualized.										
TX.1.1—Services and settings are identified and used to meet care goals.										
TX.1.1.1—There is justification for a patient need that is not addressed.										

✓ -met   ✗ -failed   ( )-comments

Figure 4.2 cont.

Medical Records Review Worksheet

Note patient record numbers.

JCAHO Standard	Record: 1	2	3	4	5	6	7	8	9	10
TX.1.2—Processes of interdisciplinary and collaborative care planning and delivery are used throughout the organization.										
TX.1.3—The patient's progress is periodically evaluated against his or her goals and the plan of care.										
TX.2.1—If anesthesia is administered, there is a care plan for anesthesia.										
TX.2.2—If anesthesia is administered, the anesthesia options and risks are discussed with the patient and/or family.										
TX.2.3—There is measurement and assessment of the physiological status during surgery.										
TX.2.4.1—Patients are discharged from postanesthesia care unit by a LIP or by using discharge criteria.										
TX.3.9—The effectiveness of medications for the patient is continually monitored.										
TX.4 —Nutrition therapy is planned.										
TX.4.1—For patients at nutritional risk, there is an interdisciplinary nutrition plan that is developed and periodically updated.										
TX.4.2—Authorized individuals prescribe or order nutrition.										
TX.4.5—The response to nutrition care is monitored.										

✓-met   ✗-failed   ( )-comments

Figure 4.2 cont.

Medical Records Review Worksheet

Record:	Note patient record numbers.									
JCAHO Standard	**1**	**2**	**3**	**4**	**5**	**6**	**7**	**8**	**9**	**10**

JCAHO Standard

TX.4.6—Special diet needs and/or altered diet schedules are accommodated.

TX.5.1.1–TX.5.1.5—Patients undergoing operative and/or invasive procedures have the following documented:
- review of patient's history,
- review of patient's physical status,
- review of diagnostic data,
- assessment of risks and benefits, and
- assessment of need to administer blood or components.

TX.5.2.1–TX.5.2.2—Operative patients have been informed about alternative options, the need for and risk of blood transfusions.

TX.5.3—Plans of care for the operative patient are documented before the procedure and should include:
- a nursing plan;
- a plan for the operative or other procedure;
- a plan for postprocedure care;
- assessment of need for additional diagnostic data;
- initial assessment of patient acuity to determine postprocedure care, and
- an initial assessment of patient's physical, mental, and neurological status and needs.

TX.5.4—Patient's postprocedure period is monitored, including:
- physiological and mental status;
- pathological findings;

✓ -met   ✗ -failed   ( )-comments

Figure 4.2 cont.

Medical Records Review Worksheet

Note patient record numbers.

JCAHO Standard	Record:	1	2	3	4	5	6	7	8	9	10
- IV fluids, drugs, and blood and components; - any unusual events or complications and their management, and - impairments and functional status.											
TX.6.1—Based on the assessment of the physical, cognitive, behavioral, communicative, emotional, pharmacological, and social needs, a treatment plan for rehabilitation patients includes at least: - patient goals for rehabilitation; - rehabilitation goals that address living, learning, and working; - measures with time frames for goal achievement; and - description of facilitating factors as well as barriers to reaching goals.											
TX.6.2—For rehabilitation patients, qualified professionals implement the rehabilitation plan with the patient and/or family, which include: - interventions to reach reasonable goals; - coordinated rehabilitation interventions; - the patient's choices, response to interventions, changes in condition, and progress toward goals; and - advocate support services to create new social support or environmental modifications.											
TX.6.3—Rehabilitation interventions improve or maintain the patient's optimal level of functioning and quality of life.											
TX.6.4—Patient is determined to end rehab services based on written discharge criteria.											

✓ -met   ✗ -failed   ( )-comments

Figure 4.2 cont.

Medical Records Review Worksheet

Note patient record numbers.

Record:	1	2	3	4	5	6	7	8	9	10

JCAHO Standard

TX.7.1—Patients placed in restraint and/or seclusion have exhausted all reasonable alternatives and have adequate justification and documentation for its use, time-limited orders for each use, and documentation that patients received attention to their needs.

TX.7.2—Patients given electroconvulsive or other convulsive therapy have adequate justification and documentation for its use, per hospital policy and procedures. Medical records of child and adolescent patients who underwent such therapy must contain the reports of two qualified child psychiatrists not directly involved in the patient's care, who have examined the patient, consulted with attending psychiatrist, and documented concurrence with the decision.

TX.7.3—Patients who had psychosurgery or other surgery for intervention of patient's mental, emotional, or behavioral disorder have adequate justification and documentation for their use.

TX.7.4 —Behavioral modification procedures and aversive conditioning have followed the hospital's policies and procedures.

TX.7.4.1—Qualified staff review, evaluate, then approve all behavioral management procedures.

Education (PF)

PF.1—Learning needs, abilities, preferences, and readiness to learn are assessed.

✓ -met   ✗ -failed   ( )-comments

Figure 4.2 cont.

Medical Records Review Worksheet

Note patient record numbers.

JCAHO Standard	Record:	1	2	3	4	5	6	7	8	9	10
PF.1.1—Learning needs assessment considers patient's cultural, religious, emotional, motivational, physical, cognitive, and language status.											
PF.1.2—Based on age and length of stay of patient, academic needs are assessed and education provided if necessary.											
PF.1.3—Patient is educated on the safe use of medication.											
PF.1.4—Patient is educated on the use of medical equipment.											
PF.1.5—Patient is educated about potential food/drug interactions, nutrition, and modified diets.											
PF.1.6—Patient is educated about rehab techniques to help him or her function more independently.											
PF.1.7—Patient is educated about additional community resources.											
PF.1.8—Patient is educated about how to obtain additional treatment, if needed.											
PF.1.9—Patient and family have been educated and are clear what their responsibilities are for the ongoing health care needs of the patient.											
PF.2—The patient education is interactive.											

✓ -met   ✗ -failed   ( )-comments

Figure 4.2 cont.

Medical Records Review Worksheet

Note patient record numbers.

Record:	1	2	3	4	5	6	7	8	9	10
JCAHO Standard										
PF.3—Discharge instructions given to the patient and/or family are also given to the organization or individual responsible for ongoing care.										
PF.4.2—Patient and family education is interdisciplinary.										
Continuum of Care (CC)										
CC.2—The entry process for the patient to a particular service reflects consideration of the appropriateness of the care, including setting and service, individualized needs, and the organization's ability to meet the needs.										
CC.2.1—Criteria define patient information necessary to determine the appropriate care setting or services.										
CC.3—The patient and family are informed about the proposed care during the entry process.										
CC.4—There is continuity of care throughout assessment, diagnosis, planning, and treatment.										
CC.5—There is coordination of care among practitioners and services.										
CC.6—CC.6.1—The patient, if referred or transferred, meets the organization's criteria for referral and transfer. Also, records of emergency patients transferred to other organizations include the reason for transfer, stability of the patient, acceptance by the receiving organization, responsibility during transfer, and follow-up planning, if required.										

✓ -met   ✗ -failed   ( )-comments

Figure 4.2 cont.

Medical Records Review Worksheet

Note patient record numbers.

Record:	1	2	3	4	5	6	7	8	9	10
JCAHO Standard										

JCAHO Standard

CC.7—Complete discharge summary exchanged when patients are admitted, referred, transferred, and discharged.

Leadership (LD)

LD.1.6—Patients with same health problems and care needs get the same quality of care throughout hospital (conscious sedation, nursing care).

LD.1.7–LD.1.7.1—Records confirm that the organization follows its approved policies and procedures on the scope of services and care provided by each department.

Management of Information (IM)

IM.7.2—Records must contain these items:
- name, address, date of birth, and legal representative;
- legal status if mental health patient;
- emergency care given prior to arrival, if any;
- conclusions or impressions from H&P;
- diagnosis or diagnostic impression;
- reasons for admission or treatment;
- diagnostic and therapeutic orders, if any;
- diagnostic and therapeutic procedures and tests and their results;
- operative and other invasive procedures performed, using acceptable terms, including etiology;

✓ -met   X -failed   ( )-comments

Figure 4.2 cont.

Medical Records Review Worksheet

Note patient record numbers.

JCAHO Standard	Record:	1	2	3	4	5	6	7	8	9	10
- progress notes by the medical staff and other authorized individuals;											
- reassessments, if needed;											
- clinical observations;											
- response to care;											
- consultation reports;											
- every medication ordered or prescribed;											
- every dose administered and any adverse reactions;											
- every medication dispensed to inpatient at discharge or to ambulatory patient;											
- all relevant diagnoses established during care;											
- any referrals/communication to other providers;											
- discharge instructions to patients and family; and											
- discharge summary containing reason for hospitalization, significant findings, procedures performed, treatment given, condition on discharge, and any instructions given to patient or family.											
IM.7.2—A final progress note may be substituted for a summary only for patients with minor problems and less than 48-hour stay, or for newborn infants or normal deliveries. Transfer summary may be used instead of discharge summary only when patients are transferred to different level of hospitalization or residential care within the organization.											
IM.7.3.1—Surgery records show preoperative diagnosis by LIP.											

✓ -met   ✗ -failed   ( )-comments

Figure 4.2 cont.

Medical Records Review Worksheet

Note patient record numbers.

JCAHO Standard	1	2	3	4	5	6	7	8	9	10
IM.7.3.2—Operative report, completed immediately after surgery, describes findings, procedure used, specimen removed, post-operative diagnosis, and name of primary surgeon and any assistants.										
IM.7.3.2.1—Operative report is authenticated and dated by surgeon.										
IM.7.3.2.2—If the operative report is not filed in medical record immediately after surgery, a progress note is entered immediately.										
IM.7.3.4—Postoperative documentation indicates discharge from PACU by an LIP or according to discharge criteria.										
IM.7.5—Records of emergency visits contain time and means of arrival.										
IM.7.5.1—Records of emergency visits contain a note if patient leaves against medical advice.										
IM.7.5.2—Records of emergency visits contain conclusions at end of treatment, including final disposition, condition, and instructions for follow-up.										
IM.7.5.3—If authorized, a copy of emergency services provided is available to practitioner providing follow-up.										
IM.7.6—Significant clinical information is entered within appropriate time frames.										

✓ -met   ✗ -failed   ( )-comments

Figure 4.2 cont.

Medical Records Review Worksheet

Note patient record numbers.

Record:	1	2	3	4	5	6	7	8	9	10

JCAHO Standard

IM.7.7—Verbal orders of authorized individuals are accepted and transcribted by qualified personnel named in the medical staff rules and regulations.

IM.7.8—All entries show author, date, and authentication, when necessary.

IM.7.9—All relevant inpatient, ambulatory care, emergency, urgent, or immediate care records are assembled and accessable when patient receives care.

Medical Staff (MS)

MS.6.1–MS.6.2.2—Only individuals privileged to admit patients and perform an H&P do so.

MS.6.2—If patient is admitted for inpatient treatment, H&P is performed by a physician privileged to do so.

MS.6.2.2.1—Records show that when LIPs provide care, physicians confirm their findings prior to major interventions.

MS.6.2.2.2—For dental patients, dentist performs part of H&P relating to dentistry.

MS.6.2.2.3—For podiatry patients, podiatrist performs part of H&P relating to podiatry.

✓ -met   ✗ -failed   ( )-comments

Figure 4.2 cont.

Medical Records Review Worksheet

Note patient record numbers.

Record:	1	2	3	4	5	6	7	8	9	10
JCAHO Standard										
MS.6.4—Records show practitioners who perform surgical or invasive procedures practice within the scope of their delineated privileges.										
MS.6.5—Records show that each patient's general medical condition is the responsibility of a qualified member of the medical staff.										
MS.6.5.2—Consultation by a physician or LIP is obtained under defined circumstances.										

✓ -met   ✗ -failed   ( )-comments

Appendix B ——————————————————————————————————— *111*

Figure 4.3

Medical Records Analysis Worksheet

JCAHO Standards	% required to score a 1	% required to score a 2	% of records with the documentation	Place a score of 1, 2, or N (non-compliance), or NA (not applicable)	Who is responsible for documenting the information?	Comments
Patient Rights (RI)						
RI.1, RI.1.2.3, RI.1.3.4—There is evidence of a resolved ethical or treatment issue.	not stated	not stated				
RI.1.1—The patient is admitted and/or transferred based on his or her need for services.	not stated	not stated				
RI.1.2—The patient and, when appropriate, the family is involved in the patient's care.	not stated	not stated				
RI.1.2.1–RI.1.3—Informed consent is obtained for treatments, or procedures, or research participants (benefits, risks, and alternatives are discussed).	not stated	not stated				
RI.1.2.2—If appropriate, surrogate decision-makers are identified.	not stated	not stated				
RI.1.2.4—The patient is asked if he or she has an advance directive, and if so, the advance directive is in the record, or the intent of the advance directive is documented.	not stated	not stated				
RI.1.2.5–RI.1.2.6—DNR and withholding or withdrawing life-sustaining treatment orders follow hospital policy.	not stated	not stated				

Figure 4.3 cont.

Medical Records Analysis Worksheet

JCAHO Standards	% required to score a 1	% required to score a 2	% of records with the documentation	Place a score of 1, 2, or N (non compliance) or NA (not applicable)	Who is responsible for documenting the information?	Comments
RI.1.2.7—The patient and family members' needs are individually addressed during the end of life.	not stated	not stated				
RI.1.3.4—Patient and/or family complaints are addressed.	not stated	not stated				
RI.1.3.5—Requested pastoral counseling is provided.	not stated	not stated				
RI.1.3.6—Individual (non-English-speaking, visually or hearing impaired) patient communication needs are considered.	not stated	not stated				
RI.2—The procurement and donation of organs and other tissues follow organizational policy.	not stated	not stated				
Assessment of Patients (PE)						
PE.1—There is a physical, psychological, and social status assessment.	90–100	75–89				
PE.1.1—The scope and intensity of further assessments are based on diagnosis, the care setting, desire for care, and response to any previous treatment.	90–100	75–89				
PE.1.2—Nutritional status is assessed when indicated by the patient's needs.	90–100	75–89				
PE.1.3–PE.1.3.1—Functional status is assessed when indicated by the patient's needs (a must for patients referred for rehab services).	90–100	75–89				

Figure 4.3 cont.

Medical Records Analysis Worksheet

JCAHO Standards	% required to score a 1	% required to score a 2	% of records with the documentation	Place a score of 1, 2, or N (non compliance), or NA (not applicable)	Who is responsible for documenting the information?	Comments
PE.1.4—Appropriate diagnostic tests are performed to determine any patient needs.	100	95–99				
PE.1.4.1—Records show requests for diagnostic tests provide adequate clinical information.	90–100	75–89				
PE.1.5—The need for a discharge planning assessment is determined.	not stated	not stated				
PE.1.6—The initial assessment is completed within the time set by hospital policy.	100	95–99				
PE.1.6.1—The H&P, nursing assessment, and other assessments are completed and recorded within 24 hours of admission for inpatients.	100	95–99				
PE.1.7—There is an H&P, indicated diagnostic tests, and a pre-operative diagnosis on the record before surgery is performed (with the exception of emergencies).	100	95–99				
PE.1.7.1—Preanesthesia assessment for patients for whom anesthesia is planned.	100	95–99				
PE.1.7.2—If anesthesia is planned, a licensed independent practitioner with appropriate clinical privileges determines if the patient is an appropriate candidate.	100	95–99				
PE.1.7.3—If anesthesia is administered, the patient is reevaluated immediately prior to anesthesia induction.	90–100	75–89				

Figure 4.3 cont.

Medical Records Analysis Worksheet

JCAHO Standards	% required to score a 1	% required to score a 2	% of records with the documentation	place a score of 1, 2, or N (non compliance), or NA	Who is responsible for documenting the information?	Comments
PE.1.7.4—The patient's status is assessed on admission to and discharge from the post-anesthesia recovery area.	90–100	75–89				
PE.1.9.1—Laboratory and pathology services and results are provided on a timely basis through the hospital's laboratories or an approved reference laboratory.	not stated	not stated				
PE.1.14.2—If patient is getting blood glucose monitored on unit, the results are traceable to the machine used for testing.	not stated	not stated				
PE.2—The patient is reassessed according to hospital policy.	not stated	not stated				
PE.2.2—Reassessment occurs at regular intervals and determines the patient's response to care.	90–100	75–89				
PE.2.3–PE.2.4—Patient is reassessed when there is a significant change in the patient's condition or diagnosis.	90–100	75–89				
PE.3—Patient needs are identified and prioritized.	90–100	75–89				
PE.3.1—Care decisions are based on identified patient needs and priorities.	90–100	75–89				
PE.4.2—For patients that need emergency care, assessments and treatment are determined by a LIP.	90–100	75–89				
PE.4.3—In areas where nursing care is provided, an RN assesses the patient's nursing care needs.	90–100	75–89				

Figure 4.3 cont.

Medical Records Analysis Worksheet

JCAHO Standards	% required to score a 1	% required to score a 2	% of records with the documentation	Place a score of 1, 2, or N (non-compliance), or NA (not applicable)	Who is responsible for documenting the information?	Comments
PE.5—Infants, children, or adolescent patients are individually assessed for psychosocial needs, development aspects, immunizations, family, or guardian expectations and involvement for treatment.	90–100	75–89				
PE.6—Emotionally or behaviorally disordered patients are individually assessed for their history of mental, emotional, behavioral, and substance abuse problems, a mental status examination, problem behaviors, and a psychosocial assessment.	90–100	75–89				
PE.7—Substance abuse patients are individually assessed for history of alcohol or drug use, physical problems associated with abuse, family history of substance abuse, spiritual orientation, previous treatment, response to previous treatment, history of physical or sexual abuse, sexual history and orientation.	90–100	75–89				
PE.8—Patients of suspected abuse or neglect are identified, appropriate consents are obtained, and legally required notifications occurred.	90–100	75–89				
Treatment of Patients (TX)						
TX.1—Records show that the care, treatment, and rehabilitation plans are appropriate and individualized.	100	95–99				
TX.1.1—Services and settings are identified and used to meet care goals.	90–100	75–89				
TX.1.1.1—There is justification for a patient need that is not addressed.	not stated	not stated				

Figure 4.3 cont.

Medical Records Analysis Worksheet

JCAHO Standards	% required to score a 1	% required to score a 2	% of records with the documentation	Place a score of 1, 2, or N (non-compliance), or NA (not applicable)	Who is responsible for documenting the information?	Comments
TX.1.2—Processes of interdisciplinary and collaborative care planning and delivery are used throughout the organization.	not stated	not stated				
TX.1.3—The patient's progress is periodically evaluated against his or her goals and the plan of care.	100	90–99				
TX.2.1—If anesthesia is administered, there is a care plan for anesthesia.	90–100	75–89				
TX.2.2—If anesthesia is administered, the anesthesia options and risks are discussed with the patient and/or family.	90–100	75–89				
TX.2.3—There is measurement and assessment of the physiological status during surgery.	100	95–99				
TX.2.4.1—Patients are discharged from postanesthesia care unit by a LIP or by using discharge criteria.	not stated	not stated				
TX.3.9—The effectiveness of medications for the patient is continually monitored.	90–100	75–89				
TX.4 —Nutrition therapy is planned.	not stated	not stated				
TX.4.1—For patients at nutritional risk, there is an interdisciplinary nutrition plan that is developed and periodically updated.	90–100	75–89				
TX.4.2—Authorized individuals prescribe or order nutrition.	90–100	75–89				
TX.4.5—The response to nutrition care is monitored.	90–100	75–89				

Figure 4.3 cont.

Medical Records Analysis Worksheet

JCAHO Standards	% required to score a 1	% required to score a 2	% of records with the documentation	Place a score of 1, 2, or N (non-compliance), or NA (not applicable)	Who is responsible for documenting the information?	Comments
TX.4.6—Special diet needs and/or altered diet schedules are accommodated.	not stated	not stated				
TX.5.1.1–TX.5.1.5—Patients undergoing operative and/or invasive procedures have the following documented: - review of patient's history, - review of patient's physical status, - review of diagnostic data, - assessment of risks and benefits, and - assessment of need to administer blood or components.	91–100	76–90				
TX.5.2.1–TX.5.2.2—Operative patients have been informed about alternative options, the need for and risk of blood transfusions.	90–100	75–89				
TX.5.3—Plans of care for the operative patient are documented before the procedure and should include: - a nursing plan; - a plan for the operative or other procedure; - a plan for postprocedure care; - assessment of need for additional diagnostic data; - initial assessment of patient acuity to determine postprocedure care, and - an initial assessment of patient's physical, mental, and neurological status and needs.	100	95–99				
TX.5.4—Patient's postprocedure period is monitored, including: - physiological and mental status; - pathological findings;	90–100	75–89				

Figure 4.3 cont.

Medical Records Analysis Worksheet

JCAHO Standards	% required to score a 1	% required to score a 2	% of records with the documentation	Place a score of 1, 2, or N (non compliance), or NA (not applicable)	Who is responsible for documenting the information	Comments
- IV fluids, drugs, and blood and components; - any unusual events or complications and their management, and - impairments and functional status.						
TX.6.1—Based on the assessment of the physical, cognitive, behavioral, communicative, emotional, pharmacological, and social needs, a treatment plan for rehabilitation patients includes at least: - patient goals for rehabilitation; - rehabilitation goals that address living, learning, and working; - measures with time frames for goal achievement; and - description of facilitating factors as well as barriers to reaching goals.	90–100	75–89				
TX.6.2—For rehabilitation patients, qualified professionals implement the rehabilitation plan with the patient and/or family, which include: - interventions to reach reasonable goals; - coordinated rehabilitation interventions; - the patient's choices, response to interventions, changes in condition, and progress toward goals; and - advocate support services to create new social support or environmental modifications.	90–100	75–89				
TX.6.3—Rehabilitation interventions improve or maintain the patient's optimal level of functioning and quality of life.	90–100	75–89				
TX.6.4—Patient is determined to end rehab services based on written discharge criteria.	90–100	75–89				

Figure 4.3 cont.

Medical Records Analysis Worksheet

JCAHO Standards	% required to score a 1	% required to score a 2	% of records with the documentation	Place a score of 1, 2, or N (non-compliance), or NA (not applicable)	Who is responsible for documenting the information?	Comments
TX.7.1—Patients placed in restraint and/or seclusion have exhausted all reasonable alternatives and have adequate justification and documentation for its use, time-limited orders for each use, and documentation that patients received attention to their needs.	90–100	75–89				
TX.7.2—Patients given electroconvulsive or other convulsive therapy have adequate justification and documentation for its use, per hospital policy and procedures. Medical records of child and adolescent patients who underwent such therapy must contain the reports of two qualified child psychiatrists not directly involved in the patient's care, who have examined the patient, consulted with attending psychiatrist, and documented concurrence with the decision.	100	95–99				
TX.7.3—Patients who had psychosurgery or other surgery for intervention of patient's mental, emotional, or behavioral disorder have adequate justification and documentation for their use.	100	95–99				
TX.7.4 —Behavioral modification procedures and aversive conditioning have followed the hospital's policies and procedures.	not stated	not stated				
TX.7.4.1—Qualified staff review, evaluate, then approve all behavioral management procedures.	not stated	not stated				
Education (PF)						
PF.1—Learning needs, abilities, preferences, and readiness to learn are assessed.	90–100	75–89				

Figure 4.3 cont.

Medical Records Analysis Worksheet

JCAHO Standards	% required to score a 1	% required to score a 2	% of records with the documentation	Place a score of 1, 2, or N (non compliance), or NA (not applicable)	Who is responsible for documenting the information?	Comments
PF.1.1—Learning needs assessment considers patient's cultural, religious, emotional, motivational, physical, cognitive, and language status.	90–100	75–89				
PF.1.2—Based on age and length of stay of patient, academic needs are assessed and education provided if necessary.	not stated	not stated				
PF.1.3—Patient is educated on the safe use of medication.	90–100	75–89				
PF.1.4—Patient is educated on the use of medical equipment.	90–100	75–89				
PF.1.5—Patient is educated about potential food/drug interactions, nutrition, and modified diets.	90–100	75–89				
PF.1.6—Patient is educated about rehab techniques to help him or her function more independently.	90–100	75–89				
PF.1.7—Patient is educated about additional community resources.	90–100	75–89				
PF.1.8—Patient is educated about how to obtain additional treatment, if needed.	90–100	75–89				
PF.1.9—Patient and family have been educated and are clear what their responsibilities are for the ongoing health care needs of the patient.	not stated	not stated				
PF.2—The patient education is interactive.	90–100	75–89				

Figure 4.3 cont.

Medical Records Analysis Worksheet

JCAHO Standards	% required to score a 1	% required to score a 2	% of records with the documentation	Place a score of 1, 2, or N (non-compliance), or NA (not applicable)	Who is responsible for documenting the information?	Comments
PF.3—Discharge instructions given to the patient and/or family are also given to the organization or individual responsible for ongoing care.	90–100	75–89				
PF.4.2—Patient and family education is interdisciplinary.	not stated	not stated				
Continuum of Care (CC)						
CC.2—The entry process for the patient to a particular service reflects consideration of the appropriateness of the care, including setting and service, individualized needs, and the organization's ability to meet the needs.	not stated	not stated				
CC.2.1—Criteria define patient information necessary to determine the appropriate care setting or services.	not stated	not stated				
CC.3—The patient and family are informed about the proposed care during the entry process.	not stated	not stated				
CC.4—There is continuity of care throughout assessment, diagnosis, planning, and treatment.	not stated	not stated				
CC.5—There is coordination of care among practitioners and services.	not stated	not stated				
CC.6–CC.6.1—The patient, if referred or transferred, meets the organization's criteria for referral and transfer. Also, records of emergency patients transferred to other organizations include the reason for transfer, stability of the patient, acceptance by the receiving organization, responsibility during transfer, and follow-up planning if required.	100	90–99				

Figure 4.3 cont.

Medical Records Analysis Worksheet

JCAHO Standards	% required to score a 1	% required to score a 2	% of records with the documentation	place a score of 1, 2, or N (non-compliance), or NA (not applicable)	Who is responsible for documenting the information?	Comments
CC.7—Complete discharge summary exchanged when patients are admitted, referred, transferred, and discharged.	90–100	75–89				
Leadership (LD)						
LD.1.6—Patients with same health problems and care needs get the same quality of care throughout hospital (conscious sedation, nursing care).	not stated	not stated				
LD.1.7–LD.1.7.1—Records confirm that the organization follows its approved policies and procedures on the scope of services and care provided by each department.	not stated	not stated				
Management of Information (IM)						
IM.7.2—Records must contain these items: - name, address, date of birth, and legal representative; - legal status if mental health patient; - emergency care given prior to arrival, if any; - conclusions or impressions from H&P; - diagnosis or diagnostic impression; - reasons for admission or treatment; - diagnostic and therapeutic orders, if any; - diagnostic and therapeutic procedures and tests and their results; - operative and other invasive procedures performed, using acceptable terms, including etiology; - progress notes by the medical staff and other authorized individuals;	90–100	75–89				

Figure 4.3 cont.

Medical Records Analysis Worksheet

JCAHO Standards	% required to score a 1	% required to score a 2	% of records with the documentation	Place a score of 1, 2, or N (non-compliance), or NA (not applicable)	Who is responsible for documenting the information?	Comments
- reassessments, if needed; - clinical observations; - response to care; - consultation reports; - every medication ordered or prescribed; - every dose administered and any adverse reactions; - every medication dispensed to inpatient at discharge or to ambulatory patient; - all relevant diagnoses established during care; - any referrals/communication to other providers; - discharge instructions to patients and family; and - discharge summary containing reason for hospitalization, significant findings, procedures performed, treatment given, condition on discharge, and any instructions given to patient or family.						
IM.7.2—A final progress note may be substituted for a summary only for patients with minor problems and less than 48-hour stay, or for newborn infants or normal deliveries. Transfer summary may be used instead of discharge summary only when patients are transferred to different level of hospitalization or residential care within the organization.	90–100	75–89				
IM.7.3.1—Surgery records show preoperative diagnosis by LIP.	100	95–99				
IM.7.3.2—Operative report, completed immediately after surgery, describes findings, procedure used, specimen removed, post-operative diagnosis, and name of primary surgeon and any assistants.	100	90–99				

Figure 4.3 cont.

Medical Records Analysis Worksheet

JCAHO Standards	% required to score a 1	% required to score a 2	% of records with the documentation	Place a score of 1, 2, or N (non-compliance), or NA (not applicable)	Who is responsible for documenting the information?	Comments
IM.7.3.2.1—Operative report is authenticated and dated by surgeon.	100	90–99				
IM.7.3.2.2—If the operative report is not filed in medical record immediately after surgery, a progress note is entered immediately.	100	90–99				
IM.7.3.4—Postoperative documentation indicates discharge from PACU by an LIP or according to discharge criteria.	not stated	not stated				
IM.7.5—Records of emergency visits contain time and means of arrival.	90–100	75–89				
IM.7.5.1—Records of emergency visits contain a note if patient leaves against medical advice.	90–100	75–89				
IM.7.5.2—Records of emergency visits contain conclusions at end of treatment, including final disposition, condition, and instructions for follow-up.	90–100	75–89				
IM.7.5.3—If authorized, a copy of emergency services provided is available to practitioner providing follow-up.	not stated	not stated				
IM.7.6—Significant clinical information is entered within appropriate time frames.	not stated	not stated				
IM.7.7—Verbal orders of authorized individuals are accepted and transcribed by qualified personnel named in the medical staff rules and regulations.	90–100	75–89				
IM.7.8—All entries show author, date, and authentication, when necessary.	90–100	75–89				

Figure 4.3 cont.

Medical Records Analysis Worksheet

JCAHO Standards	% required to score a 1	% required to score a 2	% of records with the documentation	place a score of 1, 2, or N (non-compliance), or NA (not applicable)	Who is responsible for documenting the information?	Comments
IM.7.9—All relevant inpatient, ambulatory care, emergency, urgent, or immediate care records are assembled and accessable when patient receives care.	75–89	90–100				
Medical Staff (MS)						
MS.6.1–MS.6.2.2—Only individuals privileged to admit patients and perform an H&P do so.	not stated	not stated				
MS.6.2—If patient is admitted for inpatient treatment, H&P is performed by a physician privileged to do so.	90–99	100				
MS.6.2.2.1—Records show that when LIPs provide care, physicians confirm their findings prior to major interventions.	90–99	100				
MS.6.2.2.2—For dental patients, dentist performs part of H&P relating to dentistry.	75–89	90–100				
MS.6.2.2.3—For podiatry patients, podiatrist performs part of H&P relating to podiatry.	75–89	90–100				
MS.6.4—Records show practitioners who perform surgical or invasive procedures practice within the scope of their delineated privileges.	90–99	100				
MS.6.5—Records show that each patient's general medical condition is the responsibility of a qualified member of the medical staff.	90–99	100				
MS.6.5.2—Consultation by a physician or LIP is obtained under defined circumstances.	not stated	not stated				

Figure 4.3 cont.

Medical Records Analysis Worksheet

JCAHO Standards	% required to score a 1	% required to score a 2	% of records with the documentation	Place a score of 1, 2, or N (non-compliance), or NA (not applicable)	Who is responsible for documenting the information?	Comments

Appendix C

Medical Record
Review Checklist

Medical Record Review Checklist

Instructions:
1. Please add up (total) all of the medical record forms.
2. For each item reviewed, enter the total number forms with the "item present" box checked in column A.
3. For each item reviewed, add the number found in column A to the total number of forms with the "item not present" box checked (column B). This number is the total number of records reviewed for this item.

Required information and related standard

General items	Can this information be found in the record?		
	A. Items present	**B.** Items not present	**C.** Items not applicable
IM.7.2* Existence of advance directives is determined			
Evidence of informed consent			
Discharge information includes all medications prescribed or dispensed at discharge			
IM.7.7 Verbal orders of authorized individuals are accepted and transcribed by qualified personnel named in medical staff rules and regulations			
IM.7.8* All entries in the record are dated, and authenticated, when necessary			
Entries made by house staff are countersigned per policy specified in medical staff rules and regulations			
TX.1* Treatment plans are documented			
PE.1.6.1* History & physical are completed within 24 hours of admission			

* Standards apply to all records

Required information and related standard

Can this information be found in the record?

EDUCATION	A. Items present	B. Items not present	C. Items not applicable
PF.1* The patient and/or, when appropriate, his or her family have their learning needs assessed			
PF.1.1 *When indicated*, the assessment includes consideration of: • cultural values • religious beliefs • barriers to learning (e.g., emotional, physical, and/or cognitive limitations)			
PF.1.2 When called for by the age of the patient and the length of stay, school-aged children are given the opportunity to continue their schooling			
PF.1.3 *When appropriate*, the patient and/or family is educated about the safe and efficient use of medications			
PF.1.4 *When appropriate*, the patient and/or family is educated about the safe and effective use of medical equipment			
PF.1.5 *When appropriate*, the patient and/or family is educated about diet and nutrition, including potential drug-food interactions			
PF.1.6 *When appropriate*, the patient and/or family is educated about rehabilitation techniques			
PF.1.7 *When appropriate*, the patient and/or family is educated about available community resources			
PF.1.10 *When appropriate*, the patient is educated regarding personal hygiene and grooming			
PF.4.2 The educational process was interdisciplinary as appropriate to the care plan			
PE.1* Initial screening or assessment is completed, including assessment of each patient's: * - physical status * - psychological status * - social status			

* Standards apply to all records

Required information and related standard

Can this information be found in the record?

	A. Items present	B. Items not present	C. Items not applicable

ASSESSMENT

PE.1.2* Need for nutritional assessment is determined

PE.1.3* Need for functional assessment is determined

PE.1.3.1 A functional assessment is performed for each patient referred for rehabilitation services

PE.1.5* Need for discharge planning is assessed

TX.3.9 Monitoring of a medication's effect on the patient includes assessment based on collective observations, including the patient's own perceptions of its effect

PE.6 Evaluation for psychiatric inpatients includes
- history of emotional problems/treatment
- history of substance abuse problems/treatment
- current emotional and behavioral functioning
- maladaptive or problem behaviors
- psychiatric evaluation
- mental status exam appropriate to patient's age

When appropriate, legal assessment of patient completed and entered in record

REASSESSMENT

PE.2* Each patient is reassessed:

PE.2.2 – to determine the patient's response to treatment

PE.2.3 – when there is significant change in the patient's condition

* Standards apply to all records

Can this information be found in the record?

Required information and related standard

REASSESSMENT

PE.3*   Patient needs are identified and prioritized through a coordinated, collaborative approach

PE.3.1* Care/treatment decisions are based on identified patient needs/priorities

OPERATIVE/INVASIVE PROCEDURES

PE.1.7   Pre-op H&P and diagnosis are recorded

PE.1.7.1 Pre-anesthesia assessment (e.g., risk, ASA) is documented

TX.2.1   Pre-op plan for anesthesia is recorded

PE.1.7.2 Patient is determined to be an appropriate anesthesia candidate

Determination is made by a licensed independent practitioner

TX.5.3   Prior to procedure, plan for nursing care is recorded

PE.1.7.3 Prior to induction, patient is re-evaluated for anesthesia

TX.2.3   Patient's physiological status is measured and assessed during anesthesia

TX.5.4   Post-operative monitoring of patient includes:
- physiological status
- mental status
- intravenous fluids administered
- drugs administered
- blood and blood components
- impairments and functional status
- unusual events: post-op complications/management

* Standards apply to all records

Required information and related standard

Can this information be found in the record?

Required information and related standard	A. Items present	B. Items not present	C. Items not applicable
OPERATIVE/INVASIVE PROCEDURES			
TX.2.4.1 Patient is discharged from the post-anesthesia recovery area by a licensed independent practitioner or;			
Patient is discharged from the post-anesthesia recovery area by meeting medical staff criteria			
OPERATIVE REPORT			
The operative report is documented immediately post-op			
The operative report includes, as applicable: - findings - procedures - specimen removed - post-op diagnosis - name of surgeon/assistant			
Operative report is authenticated by surgeon			
IM.7.3.2 A progress note about the operation is entered immediately when there is a transcription delay			
RESTRAINT/SECLUSION			
TX.7.1 Justification for the use of restraint and/or seclusion is documented			
A physician's time-limited order is obtained each time restraint and/or seclusion is used (order specifies start and end times)			
Patient needs are attended to in accordance with organization policy and procedures			

* Standards apply to all records

Required information and related standard

Can this information be found in the record?

AMBULATORY RECORDS	A. Items present	B. Items not present	C. Items not applicable
IM.7.4　For patients receiving continuing ambulatory care services, there is a list of the following: 　- known significant medical diagnoses and conditions 　- known significant operative and invasive procedures 　- known adverse and allergic drug reactions 　- medications known to be prescribed for and/or used by the patient			
IM.7.4.1　The list stated above is started by the third visit			
EMERGENCY			
IM.7.2　Emergency care provided to the patient prior to arrival, if any, is documented			
IM.7.5.2　Conclusions at the termination of treatment, including: 　- final disposition 　- condition at discharge 　- any instructions for follow-up care			
CC.6　Emergency patient transfers to other organizations include: 　- reason for transfer 　- stability of patient 　- acceptance by the receiving organization 　- responsibility during transfer			
CC.7　- relevant patient information goes with the patient			

* Standards apply to all records

Required information and related standard

Can this information be found in the record?

PEDIATRIC RECORDS	A. Items present	B. Items not present	C. Items not applicable

PE.5   As *appropriate*, the assessment of infants, children, and adolescents includes:
   - developmental age
   - length/height
   - head circumference
   - weight			

As *appropriate*, assessment includes consideration of the patient's education needs and daily activities			
Immunization status is recorded			
Family/guardian expectations for and involvement in the assessment, initial treatment, and continuing care of the patient are documented			

RESEARCH, EXPERIMENTATION, CLINICAL TRIALS	A. Items present	B. Items not present	C. Items not applicable
Before requesting consent for participation in research, experimentation, and/or clinical trials all patients are supplied with			
RI.1.2.1.1 - description of benefits to be expected RI.1.2.1.2 - description of potential discomforts and risks RI.1.2.1.3 - description of alternative services RI.1.2.1.4 - full explanation of procedures to be followed RI.1.2.1.5 - assurance of right to refuse to participate			

RI.3.1   All consent forms related to research, experimentation, and/or clinical trials indicate
   - name of person who supplied prospective participant with information
   - date form was signed
   - address the participant's right to privacy
   - confidentiality
   - safety			

* Standards apply to all records

Required information and related standard

Can this information be found in the record?

PATIENT RIGHTS (RESTRICTIONS)	A. Items present	B. Items not present	C. Items not applicable
RI.1.3.6.1 Therapeutic indications necessitating restrictions are evaluated for therapeutic effectiveness			
RI.1.3.6.1.1 Restrictions are explained			
Restrictions are determined with participation of patient/family			

* Standards apply to all records

Continuing Education Quiz

Continuing Education Quiz:
Information Management—
A Guide to the JCAHO Standards

Directions

- Complete the quiz by clearly writing the letter corresponding to the correct choice for each question on the answer sheet found on the last page. If you expect more than one person to take the quiz, photocopy the answer sheet and use the copy to record your responses. The answers to each question can be found in the chapters of *Information Management—The Compliance Guide to the JCAHO Standards*. You may refer to the chapters as you take the quiz.

- Send only the answer sheet back to us with a $35 payment for each person who completes the quiz. You may submit your photocopied answer sheet. To qualify for the six hours of CE credit, you must get 75% of the answers correct—that's 45 out of 60 questions.

- We'll send you a certificate of completion which you may use for display and for documentation of your CE hours for the American Health Information Management Association (AHIMA).

This test has the approval of the American Health Information Management Association (AHIMA) for six continuing education hours.

Chapter 1

1. Hospital leaders are responsible for developing an information plan and integrating it with other mandated organization-wide plans.

A. true
B. false

2. How do information management standards relate to performance improvement?

A. directly
B. indirectly
C. there is no clear connection
D. none of the above

3. To efficiently comply with JCAHO information management standards, your organization should _____.

A. create independent IM task forces in each department
B. establish a multi-department project team
C. define management strategies and policies
D. B and C

4. The team monitoring compliance with patient records standards should include _____.

A. a quality manager
B. key providers
C. users of patient information
D. all of the above

5. Which of the following is the JCAHO concerned with in regard to the patient record?

A. completeness and accessibility
B. quality and accessibility
C. security and confidentiality
D. none of the above

6. How will *Information Management—The Compliance Guide to the JCAHO Standards* assist you?

A. it will help to plan your hospital's information management agenda

B. reading it will guarantee your hospital is accredited

C. it will eliminate the need to read the *Accreditation Manual for Hospitals (AMH)*

D. all of the above

Chapter 2

1. A 60-bed hospital would most likely utilize an information system similar to that of a neighboring 250-bed facility.

A. true

B. false

2. The JCAHO's document review session _____.

A. is conducted with hospital participation

B. takes a day to complete

C. is held on the first day of a survey

D. is a series of interviews

3. To comply with the IM.1 standard, hospital leaders might, for example _____.

A. assess the costs of various technologies

B. determine the legal status for patients receiving mental health services

C. aggregate data for diagnoses and performed procedures

D. ensure medical records are completed in a timely fashion

4. Recently, JCAHO surveyors have focused most heavily on which of the following?

A. written department policies

B. interviews and observations

C. medical staff knowledge of information management

D. A and C

5. The information management standard that discusses ongoing record reviews is

_____.

A. IM.3 or the capture of data
B. IM.1 or information management planning
C. IM.8 or aggregate information
D. IM.9 or knowledge-based information

6. What does IM.1 require hospitals to do?

A. plan and reorganize information management systems
B. design information management systems around the needs of the medical staff
C. plan and design information management systems around the needs of the organization
D. plan information management systems around continuous quality

7. The transmission of information standard (IM.5) might be surveyed during which of the following?

A. medical staff and nursing leadership interviews
B. medical record interview
C. information management interview
D. all of the above

8. A patient's name, reason(s) for admission, medications ordered, and the legal status of patients receiving mental health services are all examples of _____.

A. required information of patients receiving mental health services
B. information taken from patients at registration
C. required contents of medical records
D. only A and B

9. IM.9, the standard on knowledge-based information, requires:

A. hospitals to standardize data sets, definitions, and codes
B. key people who generate, collect, and analyze data to be educated on the principles of information management
C. resources to be available to hospital staff for them to gather knowledge and maintain patient care skills
D. none of the above

10. JCAHO surveyors expect all departments of a hospital, except the medical staff, to be knowledgeable of information management.

A. true
B. false

11. Surveyors will ask to see medical record reviews for what time period?

A. the current quarter
B. the previous quarter
C. the last 4 quarters
D. the last 2 years

12. To comply with the IM.2 standard, a hospital must _____.

A. have a uniform method for data capture
B. educate staff members who participate in information management
C. prove all clinical information is confidential, secure, and safe from physical damage
D. ensure all information systems are integrated

Chapter 3

1. Which of the following is responsible for communicating the results of the information project to the governing board and medical staff?

A. working group

B. decision group

C. facilitator

D. project leader

2. Once an information plan is devised for your institution, it will never need to be revised.

A. true

B. false

3. An inventory questionnaire asks about _____.

A. reports provided to external organizations

B. automated systems' use and adequacy

C. data elements in each database

D. all of the above

4. Hospitals should have a policy addressing _____.

A. the use of computer passwords

B. confidentiality and access to sensitive information

C. who can hand out release of information forms

D. all of the above

5. Which of the following is a key initial step in any information management project?

A. determining the level of automation in an information system

B. determining how to implement the project's results

C. determining exactly how long the project will last

D. only A and B

6. To best identify future needs and uses for information, a hospital must

_____.

A. develop information project descriptions
B. consider opportunities for improvement of current systems
C. compare its information budget to the budget of a substantially larger hospital
D. A and B

7. Why does the integration strategy activity address IM.6 and IM.9?

A. it allows for medical records assessment and direction
B. it looks at the needs of the patient record
C. it addresses the need to synthesize data as well as knowledge-based systems throughout the hospital
D. documentation generated in this activity can be used to show that performance improvement activities were conducted

8. To successfully complete an information management project, you must do which of the following?

A. develop strategies
B. set priorities
C. identify future needs
D. all of the above

9. Which IM standard is met by planning a library services strategy?

A. IM.1
B. IM.7
C. IM.9
D. IM.3

10. An implementation plan contains which of the following?

A. project work plans
B. decision group input
C. schedules
D. all of the above

11. The information budget presented to the hospital governing board should not reflect concern for the hospital's financial constraints.

A. true
B. false

12. A facilitator's job is to _____.

A. set agendas
B. take all minutes at meetings
C. monitor the progress of a project
D. A and C

Chapter 4

1. The basic principle of QI is to make decisions based on _____.

A. instinct
B. data
C. perceptions
D. suspicions

2. A very important element of brainstorming is that ideas be _____.

A. written down
B. generated without thought to their logic or merit
C. applicable to the problem being addressed
D. discussed individually as they are generated

3. A flow chart _____.

  A. identifies all of the steps in a process
  B. visually represents activities within a department
  C. is similar to brainstorming, except for its use of a rating system
  D. A and B

4. The medical record proves that a hospital follows its own policies, procedures, and mission.

  A. true
  B. false

5. A decision matrix _____.

  A. determines how often an event occurs
  B. collects feedback on a system
  C. evaluates, compares, and seeks out alternative solutions to problems
  D. shows the progress of a process over time

6. An ongoing medical records review should _____.

  A. include at least one record for each physician over the course of a year
  B. include only high-risk procedures
  C. not focus on whether records comply with JCAHO standards
  D. include a sample of no more than 30 records if a hospital's discharges are between 2,000 and 5,000 per year

7. A medical records review worksheet is a way to _____.

  A. assess medical records' compliance with JCAHO standards
  B. obtain baseline data in order to make accurate decisions
  C. plot productivity in medical records departments over time
  D. only A and B

8. The group primarily responsible for assessing documentation problems is

_____.

A. documentation improvement task force
B. medical records committee
C. QI team
D. all of the above

9. The ongoing medical records review will comply with JCAHO standard IM.3.3.1 if

_____.

A. all aspects of the ongoing review are documented in reports
B. the review is conducted for completeness and accuracy
C. it examines records containing only common diagnoses
D. A and B

10. A hospital should conduct a baseline review of its records to identify the extent of its documentation problems.

A. true
B. false

11. Improved documentation will have little effect on the daily operation of a hospital or the quality of care patients receive.

A. true
B. false

12. Which of the following are examples of educational ideas to improve documentation?

A. inservices
B. special events
C. reminders in medical records
D. only A and C

Chapter 5

1. The information management interview _____.

A. is conducted on the first day of the survey
B. assesses a hospital's IM planning
C. is attended by the entire medical records staff
D. has been a key part of the survey for the past 15 years

2. Surveyors focus primarily on documentation during the information management interview.

A. true
B. false

3. An information management director should be prepared to discuss which of the following topics?

A. clinical pertinence of records
B. use of comparative data
C. information integration within the hospital
D. all of the above

4. A hospital will be well prepared for the medical record interview, if it

_____.

A. conducts rehearsal sessions
B. teaches participants how to locate items listed on the review form
C. instructs participants to review the IM-related standards
D. all of the above

5. JCAHO surveyors will question only the medical records staff about IM standards.

A. true
B. false

6. A topic about which a surveyor might question an emergency care service member is

_____.

A. the control register process
B. use of aggregate data
C. timeliness of diagnostic tests
D. how IM services meet the needs of the organization

7. What are the three main sessions during a JCAHO survey that focus on information management?

A. document review session, information management interview, medical record interview
B. medical record interview, competency review, information management interview
C. documentation review session, pharmacy interview, patient unit visits
D. information management interview, patient unit visits, competency review

8. Which of the following documents may be examined during the documentation review session for compliance with IM.7?

A. discharge information on medications prescribed and dispensed
B. a listing of external comparative databases
C. a listing of continuous power commitments for the information system
D. a plan for acquisition of application software

9. All department directors should know which of the following to prepare for JCAHO survey interviews?

A. the timeliness of diagnostic tests
B. DEA and poison control information
C. use and availability of knowledge-based information
D. how data is used for performance improvement

10. Because JCAHO surveyors may interview any hospital staff member, it is important for the staff to understand _____.

A. how the information management standards affect overall hospital functions
B. the types of aggregate data used in decision-making
C. A and B
D. none of the above

11. The hospital's survey coordinator should document information management issues raised in meetings, actions that were taken, and results achieved to prepare for the document review session.

A. true
B. false

12. Hospital staff members need to be familiar with only the IM standards related to their particular department.

A. true
B. false

Appendices

1. What does AHIMA stand for?

A. American Home Infusion Medical Association
B. American Health Information Management Association
C. American Healthcare Information Managing Association
D. American Health Inspection Management Association

2. A medical records analysis worksheet helps to identify _____.

A. the percentage of records required to score a 1
B. the percentage of records required to score a 2
C. the percentage of records with correct documentation
D. all of the above

3. What services does The Accreditation Resource provide?

A. publishes *Healthcare Information Management*
B. offers seminars on JCAHO accreditation and information management
C. publishes *Healthcare Forum Journal*
D. none of the above

4. JCAHO standard TX.6.3 requires that:

A. records show that qualified professionals implement rehabilitation plans
B. records show that patients are discharged from the program based on written criteria
C. records show that rehabilitation interventions improve or maintain the patient's optimal level of functioning and quality of life
D. records show the organization has a mechanism that addresses the use of special procedures

5. What percentage of a hospital's records must comply with standard TX.1.3 to score a 1?

A. 75%
B. 85%
C. 95%
D. 100%

6. What type of a worksheet is in Appendix B?

A. documentation review worksheet
B. medical records review worksheet
C. information management interview worksheet
D. competency review worksheet

Answer Sheet

We suggest that you photocopy this page and use the copy for your responses. Please write the letter corresponding to the correct answer next to the question numbers below.

Chapter One	Chapter Two	Chapter Three	Chapter Four	Chapter Five	Appendices
1.	1.	1.	1.	1.	1.
2.	2.	2.	2.	2.	2.
3.	3.	3.	3.	3.	3.
4.	4.	4.	4.	4.	4.
5.	5.	5.	5.	5.	5.
6.	6.	6.	6.	6.	6.
	7.	7.	7.	7.	
	8.	8.	8.	8.	
	9.	9.	9.	9.	
	10.	10.	10.	10.	
	11.	11.	11.	11.	
	12.	12.	12.	12.	

Check one: ❏ ART ❏ RRA ❏ Other (please specify) _____

Name_____ Phone _____

Address_____

City _____ State_____ Zip_____

AHIMA (AMRA) ID #_____

Please enclose a check for $35 payable to Opus Communications for each individual test being submitted. Mail to:

Opus Communications
P.O. Box 1168
Marblehead, MA 01945

Other Publications from Opus Communications

Monthly newsletters

Medical Records Briefing
Credentialing Resource Center
   - Clinical Privilege White Papers
   - Briefings on Credentialing
Medical Staff Briefing
Briefings on JCAHO
Briefings on JCAHO—Home Care
Briefings on Long-Term Care Regulations

Briefings on Practice Management
Executive Briefings on Hospital Regulation
Briefings on Assisted Living
Respiratory Care Manager
Briefings on Laboratory Safety and Accreditation
Briefings on Subacute Care
Briefings on Hospital Safety

Books, Manuals, and Monographs

Information Management—A Guide to the JCAHO Standards
Health Information Management: Challenges and Solutions
Effective Survey Preparation Workbook and Guide
Quality Improvement Techniques for Hospital Safety
Quality Improvement Techniques for Long Term Care
Quality Improvement Techniques for Medical Records
Quality Improvement Techniques for Radiology
Quality Improvement Techniques for Respiratory Care
The Credentialing Desk Reference: A Complete Listing of Primary Sources, Definitions, Hard-to-Find
   Facts, and Advice
Credentialing in the Managed Care Environment
Medical Staff Credentialing—A Guide for Developing Policies and Procedures
The Compliance Guide to the Medical Staff Standards: Winning Strategies for your JCAHO Survey
Medical Staff Leaders' Practical Guide
How to Select, Orient, and Support Physician Leaders—A Guide for Hospitals and Managed
   Care Organizations
Medical Staff Reengineering Monograph Series: Reducing the Bureaucracy (Volume 1),
   Streamlining Quality Monitoring (Volume 2), Seven Success Stories (Volume 3),
   Smaller Document, Bigger Impact: Streamlining the Bylaws (Volume 4), To the Point: Effective
   Communications for the Medical Staff (Volume 5), Credentialing Without Complexity (Volume 6)
Effective Survey Preparation for Home Care Organizations
The JCAHO and Medication Use—A Monograph on Compliance and Good Practice
How to Avoid 10 Common HCFA Deficiencies
NetPractice: A Beginner's Guide to Healthcare Networking on the Internet

For more information, contact:

Opus Communications
P.O. Box 1168
Marblehead, MA 01945
Telephone: 800/753-0131 or 781/639-1872
Fax: 781/639-2982
E-mail: customer_service@opuscomm.com

Visit the Opus Communications World Wide Web site: http://www.opuscomm.com

Order Coupon

I'd like to order more copies of *Information Management— The Compliance Guide to the JCAHO Standards.*

❏ Please send me ____ copies of *Information Management— The Compliance Guide to the JCAHO Standards* at $67 per copy.

Name & Title _____

Organization _____

Address _____

City _____ State _____ Zip _____

Telephone _____

❏ Payment enclosed.   ❏ Please bill me. PO # _____

❏ VISA   ❏ MasterCard   Card # _____ Expires _____

Signature *(required for authorization)* _____

| Telephone: 800/639-0515 | Opus Communications P.O. Box 1168 Marblehead, MA 01945 | Fax: 800/639-8511 |

Order Coupon

I'd like to order more copies of *Information Management— The Compliance Guide to the JCAHO Standards.*

❏ Please send me ____ copies of *Information Management— The Compliance Guide to the JCAHO Standards* at $67 per copy.

Name & Title _____

Organization _____

Address _____

City _____ State _____ Zip _____

Telephone _____

❏ Payment enclosed.   ❏ Please bill me. PO # _____

❏ VISA   ❏ MasterCard   Card # _____ Expires _____

Signature *(required for authorization)* _____

| Telephone: 800/639-0515 | Opus Communications P.O. Box 1168 Marblehead, MA 01945 | Fax: 800/639-8511 |

Opus Communications
P.O. Box 1168
Marblehead, MA 01945
Telephone: 781/639-1872
Fax: 781/639-2982

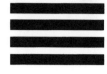

BUSINESS REPLY MAIL
FIRST CLASS   PERMIT NO 295   MARBLEHEAD, MA

OPUS COMMUNICATIONS
PO BOX 1168
MARBLEHEAD MA 01945-9939

NO POSTAGE
NECESSARY
IF MAILED
IN THE
UNITED STATES

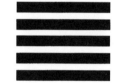

BUSINESS REPLY MAIL
FIRST CLASS   PERMIT NO 295   MARBLEHEAD, MA

OPUS COMMUNICATIONS
PO BOX 1168
MARBLEHEAD MA 01945-9939